At Work in the World

Proceedings of the Fourth International Conference on the History of Occupational and Environmental Health

Perspectives in Medical Humanities

Perspectives in Medical Humanities publishes scholarship produced or reviewed under the auspices of the University of California Medical Humanities Consortium, a multi-campus collaborative of faculty, students and trainees in the humanities, medicine, and health sciences. Our series invites scholars from the humanities and health care professions to share narratives and analysis on health, healing, and the contexts of our beliefs and practices that impact biomedical inquiry.

General Editor

Brian Dolan, PhD, Professor of Social Medicine and Medical Humanities, University of California, San Francisco (UCSF)

Recent Monograph Titles

Health Citizenship: Essays in Social Medicine and Biomedical Politics
By Dorothy Porter (Fall 2011)

Paths to Innovation: Discovering Recombinant DNA, Oncogenes and Prions, In One Medical School, Over One Decade
By Henry Bourne (Fall 2011)

The Remarkables: Endocrine Abnormalities in Art
By Carol Clark and Orlo Clark (Winter 2011)

Clowns and Jokers Can Heal Us: Comedy and Medicine
By Albert Howard Carter III (Winter 2011)

mh

www.medicalhumanities.ucsf.edu

brian.dolan@ucsf.edu

This series is made possible by the generous support of the Dean of the School of Medicine at UCSF, the Center for Humanities and Health Sciences at UCSF, and a Multi-Campus Research Program grant from the University of California Office of the President.

At Work in the World

Proceedings of the Fourth International Conference on the History of Occupational and Environmental Health

From the international conference that took place in San Francisco, CA, USA, June 19-22, 2010.

Edited by Paul D. Blanc, MD and Brian Dolan, PhD

First published in 2012
by University of California Medical Humanities Press
In partnership with the Berkeley Electroic Press and California Digital Library

Cover Photo Credit: First Aid to the Injured (Man equipped with Draeger Oxygen Helmet). Photograph by Lewis Hine, 1911. Pencil notation on reverse states: "The need for presence of these rescue outfits is a strong argument against use of boys." Gelatin silver print, collection of Paul Blanc. The image is also held in the National Child Labor Committee, Library of Congress (Lot 7477, no. 1933). This identifies the location as the Avondale Shaft, D.L.W Colliery (Pennsylvania). Print size 5 inch x 7 inch.

Library of Congress Control Number: 2011943271

ISBN 978-0-9834639-4-8

Printed in USA

Contents

Acknowledgments xii

Preface xiii

PROLOGUE

Fear and Fame
Philip Levine, Poet Laureate of the United States xviii

KEYNOTES AND COMMENTS

Keynote One
Occupation, Environment and Health: A History of Changing Perceptions and Priorities
Christopher Sellers, Stony Brook, USA 1

Comment: Occupation, Environment and Health: A History of Interdependence
Dan Berman, Davis, USA 19

Comment: Conceptualizing Hazards
Christine Meisner Rosen, Berkeley, USA 29

Comment: Air Pollution and the Meuse Valley Fog of December 1930
Benoit Nemery, Leuven, Belgium 33

Keynote Two
"An Injury to One is an Injury to All": Movements for Occupational and Environmental Health in Twentieth-Century America
Gerald Markowitz & David Rosner, New York, USA 40

Comment: Movements for Occupational and Environmental Health: History and Politics
Allison L. Hepler, Farmington, USA 56

Comment: Occupational Health Movements in France: History, Historiography and Politics
Laure Pitti, Paris, France 60

Comment: Building on the Past
Joseph Melling, Exeter, UK 64

Keynote Three
Occupatioal Disease and Labor Health and Safety Under the Nazis
Robert N. Proctor, Palo Alto, USA 68

Comment: Occupational Health under Fascism in Italy
F. Carnevale, A. Baldasseroni, S. Iavicoli, C. Petyx, L. Tomassini, Florence, Italy 84

Comment: Occupational Health in Japan During the "15 years war"
Bernard Thomann, Paris, France 89

Comment: Occupational Health in the First Francoism, 1939-1953
Alfredo Menéndez-Navarro, Granada, Spain 93

Expanded Abstracts

Occupational Health in Hippocratic Writings
H.S. Vuorinen & T.J. Hannu, Helsinki, Finland 99

Work and Disease in Greco-Roman World: Myth and Reality
M.A. Riva, V.A. Sironi, D. Fano, G.C. Cesana, Milan, Italy 102

Modern Dilemmas in Occupational Medicine and Insights from the "Hebrew Law": Nothing is New Under the Sun
Yehuda Lerman, Tel Aviv, Israel 104

Occupational Exposures and Transnational Networks in African Uranium Mines
Gabrielle Hecht, Ann Arbor, USA 108

Notions of Nature and the Debate over Vaccination in Late 20th-century US
Elena Conis, San Francisco, USA 110

Musculoskeletal Disorders: A Long Way Before Recognition, a Spectacular Course After: The French Case in the Twentieth Century
N Hatzfeld, Evry, France 113

The Ups and Downs of US Ergonomics Standards
David Rempel, San Francisco, USA 115

Work-Related Neurobehavioral Toxicity from a Historical Perspective
R Giliol, Milan, Italy & R Lucchini, Brescia, Italy 117

Harriet Hardy and the Workers of Los Alamos
Ken Silver, Johnson City, USA 120

The "Invisible" Role of the Women's Movement to the Improvement of Working Conditions at the End of the Nineteenth Century: The Case of Ersilia Majno Bronzini
Salerno Silvana, Rome, Italy & Babini P. Valeria, Bologna, Italy 123

Magic Bullet or Snake Oil? Aluminium Dust and the Prevention of Silicosis in Western Australia, 1938-1963
Criena Fitzgerald, Perth Western Australia 126

Miner's Asthma, Pneumoconiosis and the Politics of Occupational Disease in Coal Country, 1900-1970
Carla C. Keirns, Stony Brook, USA 129

Storming the Citadel: Popular Epidemiology and Scientific Innovation in British Silicosis Research
Joseph Melling, Exeter, UK 132

Grindstone City's Second Product Silicosis, the Plausibility of Export of Dust Disease
A.L. Redford, M.L. Zaremba, K.M. Elliott, S.P. Reddy, Port Huron, USA 133

Italian Workers' Health Between the Two World Wars
A. Baldasseroni, Florence, Italy, F. Carnevale, Florence, Italy, S. Iavicoli, Rome, Italy, C. Petyx, Rome, Italy, L. Tomassini, Bologna, Italy 136

Occupational Health and Safety in Australia: The International Context 1900-1939
Rod Noble, Newcastle, Australia 139

Science and Sales: Marketing the Pesticide DBCP in the Mid-Twentieth-Century United States
Susanna Rankin Bohme, Attleboro, USA 144

Tuberculosis Germs at Work: Infection, the Labour Movement and the British Workplace, c1900-1960
Arthur McIvor, Glasgow, UK 146

The Birth of the Italian Workers' Compensation Authority and its Contribution to Improving Health Conditions of Workers and General Population
G. Bonifaci, Rome, Italy, C. Sferra,Rome, Italy, M.A. Riva, Milan, Italy, M. Marchesi, Milan, Italy, V.A. Sironi, Milan, Italy 149

The History of the Workers' Compensation in Sweden
Kjell Torén & Sara Stendahl, Gothenburg, Sweden 152

Measuring Disability: Evaluating the Corporal Damage in Occupational Accident Victims and the Development of Occupational Health in Spain, 1900-1936
J. Martínez-Pérez & M. Del Cura, Castilla-La Mancha, Spain 154

The Trades Union Congress and the Politics of Industrial Health in Britain, 1920-1960
Vicky Long, Glasgow, UK 158

An Enslaved Population: The Work of Italian Military Internees (IMI) in Germany, 1943-1945
Alessandro Porro, Brescia, Italy, Bruno Falconi, Brescia, Italy, Carlo Cristini, Brescia, Italy, Lorenzo Lorusso, Chiari, Italy, Andrea Colombo, Milan, Italy, Antonia Francesca Franchini, Milan, Italy 161

Sea Fevers: The Management of Infectious Disease at Sea in the British Merchant Fleet 1867-1967
J.T. Carter, Bergen, Norway 163

The Dawning of Accident Prevention in Milan: Workers, Trade Unions, Society, 1894-1896
Falconi Bruno, Brescia, Italy, Porro Alessandro, Brescia, Italy, Lorusso Lorenzo, Chiari, Italy, Colombo Andrea, Milan, Italy, Franchini Antonia Francesca, Milan, Italy 166

The Fight Against Lead Poisoning in the Paint Industry: A Comparison of the French and American Experiences, 1900-1940
Judith Rainhorn, Paris, France 169

The Struggle for Lead Poisoning Recognition in the Workplace in France: The 1970s Turning Point
Laure Pitti, Paris, France 172

Challenging the "Blind Spots" of Expertise: Locally Produced Knowledge and Asbestos Hazard Management in Spain, 1975-1984
Alfredo Menéndez-Navarro, Granada, Spain 175

The History and Impact of Presumptive Disability Laws for Firefighters
J. A. Taylor, Philadelphia, USA, J.P. Phillips, Mississippi State, USA, B.L. Hall, St. Louis, USA 178

Abstracts

The Life and Death of Gaius Julius Caesar from an Occupational Health Perspective
Jouni J.K. Jaakkola, Oulu, Finland 183

The Discovery of the Migrant Workers by Psychiatry
Benoît Majerus, Brussels, Belgium 184

Hospitality Workers' Exposure to Secondhand Smoke from 2006 to 2008 in Beijing, China
Ruiling Liu, Berkeley, USA, Yanmin Lu, Yuan Jiang, Beijing, China 185

The Health of Sugarcane Workers in Brazil
FLR Rocha, São Paulo, Brazil, MHP Marziale, São Paulo, Brazil, OS Hong, San Francisco, USA 186

Flame Retardants, Policy, and Public Health: Past and Present
Arlene D. Blum, Berkeley, USA 188

Walt Whitman: An American Civil War Nurse who Witnessed the Advent of Modern American Medicine
D.C. Hsu, Sacramento, USA 189

The Magnificent Brown Family: Practitioners Caring for Working Women and Families, 1875-1925
Meredith Eliassen, San Francisco, USA 191

What is Worth Knowing, Experiencing and Sharing: Alice Hamilton and Contemporary Occupational Health Curricula
Leslie Nickels, Chicago, USA 192

Helmut Valentin and the Institute of Occupational Medicine in Erlangen, Bavaria
J. Richard E. Thuerauf, Erlangen, Germany 193

Working Conditions, Morbidity and Mortality at the Dutch Merchant Navy in the 17th and 18th Centuries: The Research of Arnold Leuftink
A.N. Weel, Utrecht, The Netherlands 195

Italian Workers' Health Between the Two World Wars of the 20th Century
A. Baldasseroni, Florence, Italy, F. Carnevale, Florence, Italy, S. Iavicoli, Rome, Italy, C. Petyx, Rome, Italy & L. Tomassini, Bologna, Italy 196

History of the Reporting of Occupational Disease in the Netherlands
Dick Spreeuwers, Amsterdam, The Netherlands 197

Development Process of Occupational Health Nurses in South Korea
K.J. June, Chonan-si, South Korea, G. Yi, Wonju-si South Korea, Y.M. Kim, Busan, South Korea, S.Y. Kim, Incheon, South Korea, O. Hong, San Francisco, USA 199

Medical History for Aircraft Maintainers: A Look to the Future
James W. Allen, Wilmington, USA 200

The History of Airline Medicine in the United States
Robert R. Orford, Rochester, USA 201

History of Construction Safety and Health
Knut Ringen, Silver Spring, USA 202

Prevention of Occupational Noise-Induced Hearing Loss: Past, Present, and Future
M.J. Kerr, Minneapolis, USA, O.S. Hong, San Francisco, USA, R. T. Satalof, Philadelphia, USA 203

Surviving the "Long Turn:" Overwork and Sleep Deprivation in the Early-Twentieth-Century American Steel Industry
Alana V. Derickson, University Park, USA 204

One to Five: The Remarkable Moment in Intellectual History that Created the ILO Encyclopaedia
Ilise L Feitshans, Lausanne, Switzerland 205

Creating Environmental and Occupational Health in the Twentieth Century: A journal, its Editorial Board, and the Field it Shaped
DR Smith, Ourimbah, Australia and TL Guidotti, Washington, DC, USA 206

Preliminary Explorations in the ACOEM Archives
Tee L. Guidotti, Washington, DC, USA 208

The Wieliczka Salt Mine: An Account of how Improved Workers Health Jumpstarted the Field of Speleotherapy
A.L. Redford, M.K. Zaremba, K.M. Elliott, S.P. Reddy, Port Huron, USA 209

Courting Clio: Historians and their Testimony in Products Liability Litigation
N.A. Schachtman & J.A. Vlizio, New York, USA 210

Epilogue

Speaking about the Other: On the Relevance of the Humanities to Occuptional Health
Brian Dolan, San Francisco, USA 213

Acknowledgments

THIS CONFERENCE AND CME activity was supported in part by educational grants from the following: NIOSH-CDC (Grant # 1R13OH009827-01); the International Commission on Occupational Health; the Center for Occupational and Environmental Health (University of California); and the Section on Occupational and Environmental Medicine, University of Gothenburg, Sweden.

We thank the international organizing committee: Tim Cater, PhD, FFOM, Norwegian Center for Maritime Medicine, University of Bergen, Bergen, Norway; Sergio Iavicoli, MD, PhD, Secretary General, International Commission on Occupational Health, Rome, Italy; Max Lum, EdD, MPA, Director, Office of Health Communication and Global Collaboration, NIOSH-CDC, Washington, DC, USA; Dorothy Porter, PhD, Professor of History of Health Sciences, Department of Anthropology, History & Social Medicine, UCSF, San Francisco, USA; Michele Riva, MD, Scientific Secretary, Research Center on the Hisotry of Biomedical Thought, University of Milano Bicocca, Milan, Italy; ELizabeth Watkins, PhD, Professor of History of Health Sciences, Department of Anthropology, History & Social Medicine, UCSF, San Francisco, USA.

Preface

Paul D. Blanc, Conference Chair

THE HISTORY OF occupational and environmental medicine is rich but has largely been relegated to passing notice or ignored altogether, even by clinical specialists in this field. Brief summaries of occupational and environmental medical history, when they are included in reviews or more rarely still in educational curricula, often have a limited focus on the biographical highlights of selected clinicians and researchers who have contributed to the development of this discipline. Yet as important as these biographies are, other historical factors are critical to the evolution of occupational and environmental health. First, advances in technology have played a driving role in occupational and environmental medicine that is unparalleled in other fields of health. It is true that advances in diagnostic and therapeutic modalities, from the microscope to the laser, demonstrate the powerful effect that technologic innovation can have on medical practice as a whole. But despite the role that such inventions have played in clinical care, the underlying pathologic processes of concern to practitioners have not changed because of them. Simply put, the microscope did not create illnesses due to new strains of bacteria. In contrast, technologic change continually introduces new occupational and environmental hazards, leading to evolving patterns of established diseases, as well as inducing entirely novel conditions never experienced before in human history. Second, the history of occupational and environment medicine reflects of the impact of larger social movements outside the narrow confines of medicine. Although other branches of medicine are not immune to such phenomena, occupational and environmental health concerns have tended to wax and wane secondary to societal forces. Thus, this important and underrecognized area of scholarship presents a major opportunity to advance the field by bringing together trained historians and occupational and environmental health clinicians and researchers for a creative exchange of ideas.

This was the central goal of the 4th International Conference on the History of Occupational and Environmental Health as with the three

International Conferences on this theme that preceded it: the first in Rome, Italy in 1998; the second in Norrköping, Sweden in 2001; and the third in Birmingham, England in 2007. In addition to the conferences themselves, published proceedings have helped to document and disseminate their output (Grieco A, Iavicoli S, Berlinguer G, eds. *Contributions to the History of Occupational and Environmental Prevention: 1st International Conference on the History of Occupational Prevention*, Rome, Italy; 4-6 October 1998, Amsterdam: Elsevier, 1999; Nelson MD, ed. *Occupation Health and Public Health. Lessons from the Past-Challenges for the Future*, 2006: Arbete och Hälse [Ventenskaplig Skriftserie], National Institute for Working Life, Sweden.

The 4th International Conference on the History of Occupational and Environmental Health was the first in the series to take place outside of Europe. It was made possible through the educational grants of a number of organizations and by the work of an international organizing committee noted in the acknowledgements (with particular thanks to my conference co-chair, Michele Riva of Milan). The conference was noteworthy in a number of ways. In addition to the superb program of scientific presentations documented in these proceedings, a pre-conference practical training workshop provided non-historians exposure to leading experts. This workshop covered basic methods and oral history-taking in occupational health (both led by Ronnie Johnston from Glasgow Caledonian University and Arthur McIvor form the University of Strathclyde); the nuts and bolts of archival research (led by Dorothy Porter and Lisa Mix of UCSF); and biographical methods (led by Barbara Sicherman, an Alice Hamilton scholar and Professor Emerita from Trinity College, Connecticut). Another highpoint was the closing reception for the conference, which took place at the library of the University of California San Francisco. This was hosted jointly by: the Program in History and Philosophy of Science and Technology, Stanford University; the Office for Science and Technology, UC Berkeley; the Medical Humanities Consortium through the Department of Anthropology, History and Social Medicine, UCSF; and the Division of Occupational and Environmental Medicine, UCSF. The reception included a special exhibition of key texts in the history of occupational medicine held in the UCSF collection, curated by Lisa Mix. The list of titles included is an apt way to conclude these introductory comments:

Agricola, Georg, 1494-1555. Georgius Agricola De Re Metallica, / tr. From The 1st Latin Ed. Of 1556, With Biographical Introduction, Annotations And Appendices... London, The Mining Magazine, 1912

Chadwick, Edwin, Sir, 1800-1890. Report on the sanitary conditions of the labouring population of Great Britain. A supplementary report on the results of a special inquiry into the practice of interment in towns. Made at the request of Her Majesty's principal secretary of state for the Home department, by Edwin Chadwick, esq., barrister at law. London, Printed by W. Clowes and sons for H. M. Stationery office, 1843

Hamilton, Alice, 1869-1970. Industrial Poisons in the United States. New York, Macmillan, 1925

Hill, Leonard, Sir, 1866-1952. Caisson sickness and the physiology of work in compressed air. London, Arnold, 1912

Nightingale, Florence, 1820-1910. Notes on nursing for the labouring classes. London, Harrison, 1868

Oliver, Thomas, Sir, 1853-1942. Diseases of occupation from the legislative, social, and medical points of view. London, Methuen & co., 1908

Pringle, John, Sir, 1701-1782. Observations on the diseases of the army. By Sir John Pringle, baronet ...London, W. Strahan [etc.] MDCCLXXV 7th ed., rev. and corrected

Ramazzini, Bernardino, 1633 1714. De Morbis Artificum. The following editions were included: 1700 – 1st edition; 1705 – 1st English edition; 1713 (2nd Italian, expanded)

James, Robert, 1705-1776. Health preserved, in two treatises. I. On the diseases of artificers / ... By Bern. Ramazini ... II. On those distempers, which arise from particular climates ... London, 1750

Patissier, Philibert, 1791-1863. Traité des maladies des artisans: et de celles qui résultent des diverses professions / d'après Ramazzini ... Paris: Baillière, 1822

Stockhausen, Samuel, 1619-1656. Libellus de lithargyrii fumo noxio morbificio ... Die Hütten Katze oder Hütten Rauch ... Die Bergsucht oder Berg-Kranckheit .. Goslariae, typis Nicolai Dunckeri, 1656

Thackrah, Charles Turner, 1795-1833. The effects of arts, trades, and professions, and of civic states and habits of living, on health...London, Longman, Rees, Orme, Brown, Green, & Longman, 1832

Trueta, Joseph, 1897-1977. Treatment of war wounds and fractures: with special reference to the closed method as used in the war in Spain / by J. Trueta, with a foreword by H. Winnett Orr. New York, Hoeber, 1940

Vernon, Horace Middleton, 1870-1951. Industrial fatigue and efficiency / by H.M. Vernon. London, G. Routledge, 1921

Volkmann, Richard von, 1839-1889. Beiträge zur Chirurgie anschliessend an einen Bericht über die Thätigkeit der chirurgischen Universitätsklinik zu Halle im Jahre 1873 / von Richard Volkmann Leipzig, Breitkopf und Härtel, 1875

Selections from the Daniel Berman papers, including the manuscript of Death on the Job. (Daniel Berman is an independent historian living in northern California and was a participant in the conference; he first published Death on the Job in 1978. An appreciation 20 years later published in New Solutions, Michael Lax noted, "Death on the Job, written by Daniel Berman in the late 1970s, inspired and informed the worker-based occupational safety and health movement.")

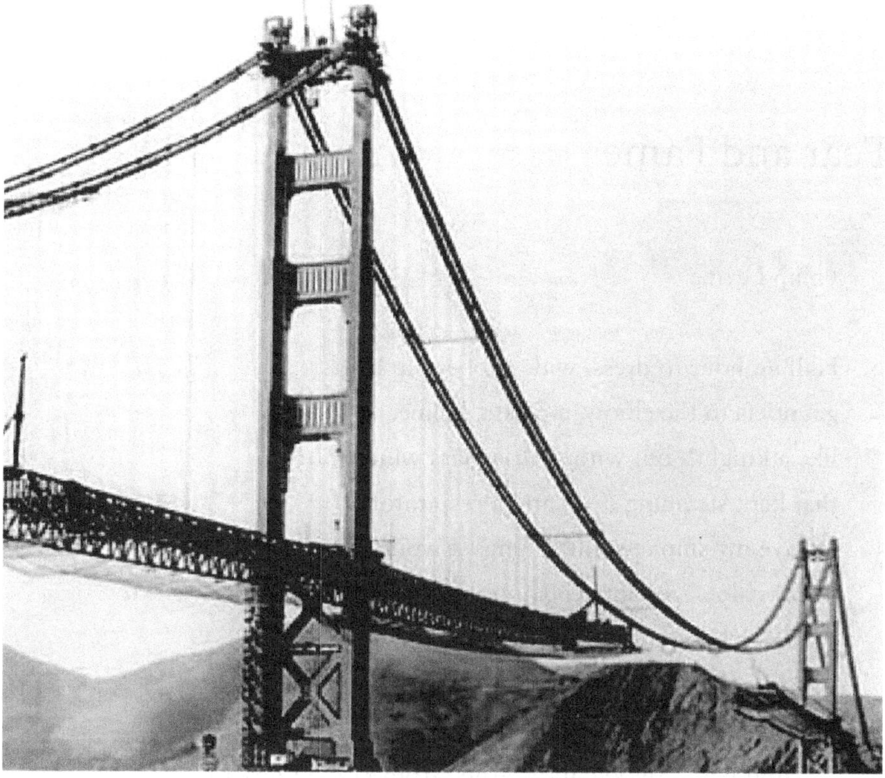

Golden Gate Bridge deck hung from cables while under construction. photographic print: b&w. 20 x 21 cm. (7 3/4 x 8 1/4 in.) 1965
Newscopy: "IT WAS A JOB MAKING BOTH ENDS MEET - Remember this? Bethlehem Steel Corp, relives the making of the Golden Gate bridge with a color movie including this scene showing iron workers hanging the roadway from steel cables. The film, a remake of a black-and-white classic, is offered to engineering groups and others free."
Courtesy San Francisco Public Library.

Fear and Fame

Philip Levine

Half an hour to dress, wide rubber hip boots,
gauntlets to the elbow, a plastic helmet
like a knight's but with a little glass window
that kept steaming over, and a respirator
to save my smoke-stained lungs. I would descend
step by slow step into the dim world
of the pickling tank and there prepare
the new solutions from the great carboys
of acids lowered to me on ropes - all from a recipe
I shared with nobody and learned from Frank O'Mera
before he went off to the bars on Vernor Highway
to drink himself to death. A gallon of hydrochloric
steaming from the wide glass mouth, a dash
of pale nitric to bubble up, sulphuric to calm,
metals for sweeteners, cleansers for salts,
until I knew the burning stew was done.
Then to climb back, step by stately step, the adventurer
returned to the ordinary blinking lights
of the swingshift at Feinberg and Breslin's
First-Rate Plumbing and Plating with a message
from the kingdom of fire. Oddly enough
no one welcomed me back, and I'd stand
fully armored as the downpour of cold water

rained down on me and the smoking traces puddled
at my feet like so much milk and melting snow.
Then to disrobe down to my work pants and shirt,
my black street shoes and white cotton socks,
to reassume my nickname, strap on my Bulova,
screw back my wedding ring, and with tap water
gargle away the bitterness as best I could.
For fifteen minutes or more I'd sit quietly
off to the side of the world as the women
polished the tubes and fixtures to a burnished purity
hung like Christmas ornaments on the racks
pulled steadily toward the tanks I'd cooked.
Ahead lay the second cigarette, held in a shaking hand,
as I took into myself the sickening heat to quell heat,
a lunch of two Genoa salami sandwiches and Swiss cheese
on heavy peasant bread baked by my Aunt Tsipie,
and a third cigarette to kill the taste of the others.
Then to arise and dress again in the costume
of my trade for the second time that night, stiffened
by the knowledge that to descend and rise up
from the other world merely once in eight hours is half
what it takes to be known among women and men.

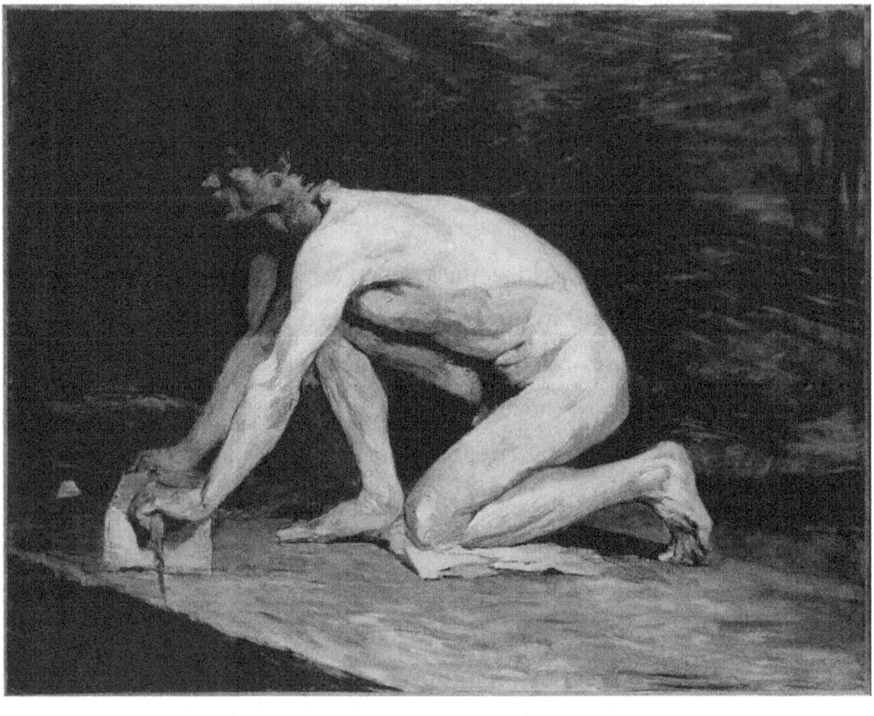

Marble Polisher: Princeton University Art Museum. Gift of the Forbes Magazine Collection: Malcolm S. Forbes, Class of 1941, Malcolm S. Forbes Jr., Class of 1970, and Christopher Forbes, Class of 1972. photo: Bruce M. White. 1882-7m. Original oil on canvas, 65.5 x 81.3 cm. Used with permission.

Keynote

Occupation, Environment and Health:
A History of Changing Perceptions and Priorities

Christopher Sellers, M.D., Ph.D.
Associate Professor of History
Stony Brook University, New York, USA

In today's America, the media gives occupational hazards short-shrift compared to its coverage of threats to the larger environment. The reporting on British Petroleum's Gulf of Mexico debacle served up yet another reminder. Of course, the first stage in this disaster was a blow-out of the Deepwater Horizon rig some 50 miles off the Louisiana coast, when eleven workers went missing and were presumed dead. The initial article covering this event appeared April 22, 2010, on page A23 of the *New York Times*. Over the ensuing days, as the leakage of underwater pipes became ever more undeniable, the spreading slick of oil itself evolved into the dominant theme of the *Times* coverage. The first time that the Gulf oil spill surged onto the front page came three weeks later. While this story was about the workers whose lives had been lost, preceding it were twenty-two articles more fixated on the looming spill itself, following its surge through the ocean and onto beaches. The *Times*' intermittent attention to these workers and their families was exceptional. For other major American newspapers, the story of the oil spill itself was what first promoted the BP disaster to the front page.[1] More captivating than grieving widows, for so many journalists, were the dying pelicans.

Now I don't mean to downplay the power of this kind of image, of oil-choked birds, nor the many other ecological dimensions of this disaster, historically unprecedented as these were. These, too, are worth caring about; I want to suggest that those of you who may be scoffing at such imagery, as peripheral to your historical and professional interest, might do well to think again. Among other reasons, it is through this kind of image that so many in our society who are not health professionals have long visualizing impending threats to their own and other peoples' bodies, in the face of expert dismissal. At the same time, it also seems clear to me these images held a greater fascination for journalists as well as environmentalists than did this disaster's first chapter, of an exploded oilrig.

Among those whose approach to industrial hazards, some hundred years earlier, stood in stark contrast, was Alice Hamilton. The pioneering American industrial hygienist did notice this kind of ecological impact, for instance, in her investigation of plants established during World War I, for making picric acid and nitrocellulose. She writes of being aided in locating these plants by "the great clouds of yellow and orange fumes, "like the pillar of cloud by day that guided the children of Israel."[2] But there was a key difference in the ways that Hamilton read the impacts of this cloud. For Alice Hamilton in 1910's America, this pollution pointed beyond itself, to the damage being wrought on workers inside these plants.

Today my goal is to trace how Americans' readings of the hazards imposed by industry have changed between Alice Hamilton's time and our own. From this standpoint, American society, like those of many other developed nations, has come a long way since Alice Hamilton's time, roughly the same period as the founding of ICOH itself. There has been an apparent evolution of spatial priorities, in which industrial hazards outside the workplace have come to seem far more spectacular and troubling than those to workers within. Holding my paper together is some media analysis, of just what makes headlines at a given time. But by also looking at, among other things, the local history of one particular smelter, I also suggest that much more is at work than just the priorities of journalists.

Now before I get too far, let me just acknowledge one contributing factor to the change: compared to early twentieth century, working conditions in the United States are now much safer and healthier. Even the worst accidents we have, in our mines or from fires, kill only a dozen workers, as opposed to the hundreds they used to. But it is an open question just how appropriate this prioritizing is, when workers may still die by the hundreds in a place like China, where so many of our goods are now made. As the ecological impacts of industry go, it remains less clear which period was worst. We have heard much hear a lot about how the Gulf Oil spill is the worst oil spill in U.S. history, at least in the sheer volume of oil released into the Gulf. And historians would be hard put to come up with an earlier human impact that comes anywhere near the scale of global climate change. Arguably, however, our ecological impacts have achieved this immense a scale precisely through our success at contending with earlier, more localized environmental devastation. And for those who lived nearby, this destruction was at least as thorough-going--and more deadly. It has become difficult for us to imagine just how ecologically catastrophic as well as dangerous the early oil fields and refineries in our own nations were, not to mention out industrial cities of the nineteenth century.

Today, however, I mean to set aside issues of any quantitative changes in workplace and local versus wider ecological impact. My starting premise is merely this: that both kinds of hazards have been present all along. Given the nature of the industrial enterprise, its dangers to workers and to an overarching ecology beyond are inherently interdependent, often linked. What has changed, in the space of relatively short, hundred plus year time space, is just how our society perceives and prioritizes these different realms of hazard over against one another. My goal is more to characterize a century-long drift in how this balance between the workplace and larger environmental impacts of industry has itself been seen and assessed in the United States.

Such a study of changes in perceptions can benefit from a common framework of analysis, one that enables us to place dissimilar experiences across many different times and places on the same analytical page. For such a purpose, discussions and findings over the last few years by an international group of scholars, many of them in attendance at this conference, have converged upon the notion of an industrial hazard regime. Industrial hazard regimes are those social arrangements, formal as well as informal, by which public bodies, private interests, and civic mobilizations handle the danger and damage associated with an industry.[3] As we have defined it, the concept is social and political, but also not just a matter for social scientists. It entails scrutiny of the variety of physical or material realms in which an industry might have posed hazards: inside workplaces, through occupational risks; outside them, through pollution and other ecological impacts; and via stores and other market exchange, as dangers to consumers. It helps, in other words, to use today's knowledge about how extensive such hazards can be to try and track their past. The nature of the historical changes we are studying makes it imperative that we consider not just those hazards that were recognized in a given time and places, but also those which went unrecognized, or under-addressed, of which we have later become aware.

Bring this concept into interplay with some media analysis, I want to suggest trends in national public attention to industrial hazards over the last century in the United States. Let me make clear at the outset the somewhat restricted definition of "public attention" on which my generalizations are based. I mean: what shows up in the text of news articles especially in the national newspaper of record for this period, the New York Times, also what federal authorities, in particular, see fit to study and perhaps regulate. These sorts of public attention to industrial hazards have gone through three distinct phases in the United States. Early on, a narrower, workplace-centered notion prevailed. Later on, industrial pollution gained in prominence. Lastly, starting in this same era but gathering steam more recently, the public face of pollution has become detached from sites of production altogether. What I want further to suggest today is that each era has added layers to our nation's overall industrial hazard regime, widened its formal scope. Each phase has had its own versions of novelty and spectacle. By the same token, in adding new varieties of expertise and control to our industrial hazard regime, each phase has also ushered in characteristic patterns of public oversight or neglect.

Writing about the history of industrial hazard regimes of necessity challenges what many of you, based on Paul Blanc's conference announcement, may take this kind of history to be. A history of industrial hazard regimes approaches the past not just for people to admire, but for larger patterns to analyze, and outcomes to critique. Rather than a series of isolated and heroic individuals, more or less like us, it demands we devote more time and thought the environment in which each operated. The social and political contexts are crucial—I will not be the last of your speakers to say so. What I want to emphasize a bit more today is the import of also attending to wider physical realms within which the experts of a given time and place operated, the more dispersed impacts of industry on its environments that contemporary experts themselves could well miss. Here is where the contemporary skills of many of you, as scientific practitioners yourselves, may well stand us historians in better stead. Analyzing the hazards of a given, past time, extrapolating from today's knowledge, we may gain a clearer picture of what a given regime did not encompass, of the kinds of hazards made more visible by regime changes later on.

As many of you are aware, it is actually around the time of Alice Hamilton, in the late nineteenth and early twentieth century, that occupational health began taking shape as an profession, first in European nations such as Germany and Britain, then in the US. This period was when the biographic approach to the field's history also began to be invented, as early practitioners sought out longer and deeper precedents for their work. There is no better illustration of just what kinds of reductions were involved in this field's invention, across many of the Western developed nations, than the discovery that the Italian doctor Bernardino Ramazzini was its father.[4]

Ramazzini as you all doubtless know, was the author of *Diseases of workers*, the first book-length treatise devoted solely to occupational factors in illness. What his biographers quickly discovered was that Ramazzini thought this book among the lesser of his own works. Prior to writing this book, during the twenty years he lived and worked in Modena, Italy, he took special pride, instead, in his work on the purity of groundwater supplies, meterology, correlating epidemics with climate and so on. His professed allegiance to a century's old classical author, Hippocrates, author of *Airs, Waters, and Places*, was so profound that Hippocrates remains the most oft-quoted author in the Morbis. As some more recent commentators have noted, these studies of the non-workplace environment actually made Ramazzini as much a processor to more broadly ecological and environmental sciences of health of the present day. Yet what drew the eyes and minds of those poised at the beginning of industrial medicine as a profession, was precisely that work in which he parted ways with the Hippocratic precedent. "When you come to a patient's house, you should ask him what sort of pains he has, what caused them, how many days he has been ill, whether the bowels are working and what sort of food he eats... I may venture to add one more question: what occupation does he follow?"[5] In the America of the early twentieth century, the time was ripe for addressing just such question, as something new. So went Alice Hamilton's early messages to her fellow doctors as well.

What Alice Hamilton and her generation saw as their own "pioneering" was, in terms of industrial hazard regimes, just one part of a larger transition from one regime toward another. It happened especially in those nations where manufacturing and heavy industry were on the rise. Germany and Britain came earliest, with US bringing up the rear—much the same order in which experts from each began attending meetings of ICOH.[6] What created these new openings and possibilities, was, to be sure, the actual hazards created by expanding industries in each nation. Yet it is also essential more clearly to recognize what these new experts themselves were more apt to downplay, namely, how much their own offices and powers owed to rising mobilizations of workers themselves. Without this kind of pressure, it is impossible to imagine the many new public interventions in the workplace of this era: new laws for compensation, as well the expanding system of factory inspection in each of these nations. Part and parcel of these transformations was the fascination they stirred in the nation's media. Newspapers and magazines, in seeking out the spectacular among workers' ills, made it all the easier to imagine that "the labor problem" was the nation's most overriding concern.

Innovators like Alice Hamilton nevertheless harbored some ambivalence toward all this attention. On the one hand, this kind of headline stirred the interest of Hamilton and her generation in problems that were specific to the workplace, as well as cultivating the creation of those positions they came to occupy. On the other hand, they also insisted that greater expertise, i.e., their own, would provide a better attack on the problem. They were challenging a neglect not only by physicians, but by managers and workers, also by the many state factory inspection outfits. Hence, while many of their inspector-predecessors, trained mostly on the job, concentrated on causes of accidents, Hamilton and her ilk sought out industrial diseases. Especially prior to the establishment of clinics and institutions in the American academy, during the 1910's, they drew especially on the European literature to claim expertise.[7]

Starting in 1910, Hamilton's career landed her at some of the institutional peaks that emerged as this new regime of workplace hazards gradually took shape. Among these, she was appointed as the first medical investigator at the federal Bureau of Labor. She thereby personified a federal presence that was quite unusual for the United States of this period, when all other charge of health matters lay with cities or states. As a federal investigator of workplace ills, she certainly had her hands full, from the cases she discovered of nitrous fume poisoning at this New Jersey munitions factory, to the high rates of lead poisoning she was able to document in so many other industries. Through such studies by her and others, in new posts in government, academia and private corporations, as well as the mounting pressures of labor unions, workers compensation not only became law in many states, but was extended to occupational diseases. But as noted at the outset, neither these experts nor the new lobbying and laws dealt with the damage from these same factories' pollution, beyond their doors.

Not that these effects were unremarkable, and even dramatic. She recognized how, outside this New Jersey munitions factory, trees nearby that had "blackened and withered," or a "sluggish stream turning the earth into something poisonous and killing the roots of all green things." But she made no systematic investigation of these consequences; nor did they even appear in any of her reports. We only know of them through her autobiography, published in 1943. But when she undertook her tour of this munitions plant, in the early 1910's, no one in the US federal government was undertaking studies of industrial water pollution, not to mention that of air.[8] Not to say these problems failed to stir much local concern especially in many of the nation's cities. But these problems, unlike those in the workplace, did not yet occupy health researchers in the federal government. Studies of oil, factory and other industrial wastes by the Public Health Service would begin in earnest in the 1920's, those of air pollution only after World War II. Until then, what research as well as enforcement was done lay in the hands of state or local health departments. [9] Compared to the attention devoted to worker hazards, industry-derived air and water pollution lay further down the list of media priorities.

Now "pollution" itself did have a more substantial currency in this time, but mostly connected with human sewage. Even though state local and local health department were gaining rapidly in legal and scientific authority over water at this same time, they themselves helped foster a certain complacency toward industrial effluents. Consider for example the water pollution discovered in the harbor of a city on the leading edge of this public health revolution, New York. In 1908, "a coating of sewage and factory waste [was discovered to have] formed over the bottom of New York Harbor." In many places several feet thick, and "gradually growing," it had "polluted the water to such an extent that thousands of fish in the Aquarium have died last year." But many public health experts, leaning on the newfound science of bacteriology, down-played the health dangers, so no typhoid or other dangerous bacillus were discovered in the wastes. Despite the deadly effects on fish, the president of the Metropolitan Sewage Commission was forced to concede that, "we have very little evidence of increase in disease from the polluted conditions of harbors." Nor had other Boards of health been able to accomplish much along this front "except where local conditions here and there become intolerable. Officers are usually unable to enforce existing laws and juries will not convict."[10]

Gradually, if more slowly than in the case of workplace dangers, a new health department-centered regime also began taking shape over the 1920s and 30s for industrial pollution. That is to say, coverage of waterborne wastes, of industry by the national industrial hazard regime in America began catching up. Hazards inflicted by industries upon consumers, as well, gained more federal attention, as a consumer movement pushed more regulation by the Food and Drug Administration and other agencies. But what is often left out, both in these and other familiar stories of an expanding regime of federal control, is just how regionally confined it tended to be. National that it purportedly was, its most thorough coverage, where federal, state and local authority more effectively intermeshed, came in the states of the northeast and midwest. We gain a still deeper understanding of just how limited the national industrial hazard regime of this period remained by also looking at the confrontation with comparable hazards in a more southerly locale, where state as well as the economy remained closer to those in the developing world.

Few lead smelters were less seen by the American state and its professional companions than one built in 1887 just outside El Paso, Texas, by Phelps Dodge. Taking advantage of lead mines in northern Mexico, it lay not a hundred yards from the Mexican border, just across the river from the Mexican town of Cuidad Juárez. Although Alice Hamilton visited smelters in Arizona and Missouri, she did not travel as far as this most "remote" of American smelters. It seems likely that Phelps Dodge workers in El Paso were like those found in the Missouri smelter Hamilton did visit: "full of malaria, hookworm, and silica dust, from the chat heaps, to say nothing of lead." Throughout the first half of the twentieth century, the state in which it arose had no workers' compensation coverage for lead poisoning.[11] The continued exclusion of this El Paso smelter from regulatory regimes that were standard in other American states suggests an intra-national and regional race to the bottom that anticipated the cross-national migrations of industrial hazards later on.[12]

Now few industrial operations of the period were as liable to impose occupational and pollution hazards as were lead smelters. But even a cursory look not just at this but at many other of the more rural industrial locations in this period also throws light on more general working assumptions among the American industrial hygienists of this period about a certain level and style of urbanization. In Chicago, where Hamilton began her work, a city health department tackled issues of sanitation, housing and sewage, not to mention smoke, justifying industrial hygiene's confinement to factory interiors. But along the Mexico–US border, a place like "Smeltertown" right beside the El Paso smelter was subject to a steady barrage of lead and other fumes from its smokestack with little or no intervention from any local health officer. We know from later studies that exposure in and around these homes could easily reach those in many parts of the plant.[13]

To return to an earlier point, we can't very well rely on biography, on the heroic vision of any Hamilton or any other occupational health practitioner, to understand the historical experience of hazard in and around this smelter. Historical reconstruction is more in order. Here, today's knowledge may aid a great deal: about just how lead travels through the environment, and affects the body, chronically as well as acutely. Doing sedimentary samples from a river next door, like the Rio Grande next to this smelter, would provide some hard evidence about the quantitative changes. But the information provided by non-medical observers at the time, or years later, can also shed light.

During the smelter's early decades, locals recollected having trouble seeing through glasses, "between coyote hair and smoke from the smelter and sand." With no baghouses to harness the fumes and particulates, "unfiltered smoke with its valuable burden of fine ores escapes from the smoke stacks." Not only must the health toll both on locals in the smelter and surrounding residents and farmers have been considerable, the sulfur dioxide in particular damaged local crops and lawns. But as late as 1938, smelter officials reported never having been sued for damages by a farmer. Instead, they adopted a practice of settling out of courts. A team from the smelter was charged with inspecting local farms and gardens for SO2 effects and paying a corresponding fee, which by 1938 added up to some $15,000.[14] Not until after World War II would the local authorities become more involved, in part because the smelter itself lay outside El Paso's city limits.

Stepping back once again to the national scale, how then did things change? How in America's culture and its public spheres, did environmental pollution trade places with workplace hazards? A long story, but one that we can make shorter by reflecting on events around 1970, the first Earth Day in the US. By this time, public concern about pollution had reached a high-water mark, historically speaking. A Gallup poll found it America's number one problem, surpassing even the war in Vietnam.[15] Congress was in the midst of thorough-going federalization, both of air and water pollution control, and of occupational health standards. Already by this time, however, the reversal had been largely accomplished, at least as far as the media was concerned. Consider this chart of mentions of pollution in the New York Times, alongside another of mentions of occupational hazards.

Why such a dramatic shift? Some commentators like to point to Rachel Carson's *Silent Spring* as starting it all, but to do so is to fall back on heroic biography and miss the deeper changes that were afoot. First we must recognize the ongoing changes in what diseases killed Americans. The United States had undergone what demographers term an epidemiological transition: tolls of mortality as well as morbidity from infectious diseases like typhoid plummeted. The chronic degenerative diseases that replaced them as the main killers of Americans, cancer and heart disease required new kinds of science to discern their causes. At the same time, environmental causality did not seem quite as forthcoming for these ailments, as it had, say for typhoid. New scientific and professional vantage points were arising as well: as the federal government increasingly funded and undertook research into environmental health, researchers began enjoying a newfound independence from corporate sponsorship. But our El Paso case study also suggests the importance of challenges not just to industry-sponsored research but to state-based industrial hygienists, and their ways of assessing environmental hazards.

Industrial hygiene, whether of the sort Hamilton had practiced in the 1910's or of that which she had preached from the Harvard School of Public Health subsequently, had a delayed arrival in El Paso. Only just after World War II did Texas legislature finally agree to begin compensating workers for occupational disease.[16] It thereby adopted a state-based legal and regulatory system that had been set up decades earlier in states such as New York and Massachusetts. Texas was thereby adding to this system of intra-workplace regulation at the margins (another way was, as in the case of black lung, by getting more and more occupational diseases officially recognized). By the 1940s and 50s, even as manufacturing continued to expand and as unionization of the American workforce approached its peak, disputes over occupational hazards now proceeded more quietly than they had. Confined to administrative channels and to a settled version of expertise, they had become much easier to keep out of the public eye. Hence, ASARCO's El Paso plant modernized its industrial hygiene program, through advice of Philip Drinker, Hamilton's Harvard colleague, there was no local publicity.[17] Neither this development, nor any mention of occupational lead poisoning, found its way into the El Paso newspaper.

Where the industrial hygienists did begin to show up in El Paso newsprint after WWII was in their discussions of local air pollution. They were the first public officials to begin measuring air pollutants in El Paso; and perpetually emphasized how discomforts of pollution did not entail any health dangers.[18] Understanding what had happened to this relationship after World War II thus requires a good deal of digging the pollution side of the story, beyond the realm of experts themselves. One direction leads into industrial change itself: for instance, into entire new classes of synthetic chemicals, from DDT to detergents, had toxic or other properties that were tailored, or turned out, to last. But as El Paso story suggests, the pollutants could be of an older sort as well. Another takes us into those new popular movements whose rising organization and clout created all these new openings for scientists and health professionals, for environmentalism and consumer protection. Looking at El Paso's history, we may also discern the bases for this new concern in other on-going environmental change. After the war, even as manufacturing jobs peaked as a percentage of the American workforce, the prospect of lives apart from factories dangled ever more insistently for widening segments of American society.

Let us look, for instance, at the continuing local history of this El Paso smelter, in connection with the city to which it was joined. After World War II, production at this smelter reached new peaks. At the same time, trends in the larger county where the El Paso smelter was located point to widespread changes in urbanization that facilitated the avoidance of polluted areas: it had become possible to live as well as work at a comfortable, more salubrious remove from such industrial plants. Over the post-war period, the well-to-do inhabitants of El Paso moved away from the factory area. Smeltertown itself came to be inhabited by mainly lower income families of Hispanic origin, whose breadwinners dominated the smelter's workforce. Those moving to the suburbs were mostly wealthy and white, and unlikely to do smelter work (Figure 4). The new public support for a more precautionary approach to pollution, here as elsewhere, reflected an evolving urban geography in the post-Second World War United States. At least for some, a group defined by differences not just in living quarters but in ethnicity or race, occupation and wealth, the possibility now boded of total escape from the factory.[19]

Now in a place like El Paso, industrial pollution also denied it. Despite what were purportedly the best efforts of the firm's hygienists, the smelter's smoke and fumes found their way into the whiter and wealthier suburbs. Their residents helped vote Bert Williams into office as the city's new mayor, in 1971, upon a campaign promise of actually taking on ASARCO, over the pollution issue. He and his associates in the health department, and then the legal department, began turning up the heat on ASARCO, with studies and then a lawsuit. The local battle they initiated, with ASARCO aligned experts then led to calls to bring in federal experts. In came a team headed by Dr. Philip Landrigan, from the Centers for Disease Control in Atlanta. The Landrigan team's study demonstrated widespread environmental contamination around the factory site, and also documented the levels and effects in neighboring children.[20]

It is remarkable, especially as compared with the controversies over lead poisoning in the early twentieth century, just how little occupational hazards figured into this early 1970's row over ASARCO's lead smelter in El Paso. The president of the smelter union, a local of the United Steel Workers, did declare "the ASARCO workers [to be] 100 per cent behind control of pollution of all kinds in El Paso," and "also obviously in favor of healthy working conditions in the ASARCO plant." And in 1975, in actuality, average lead levels in this ASARCO operation were considerably higher than in its smelters in other parts of the US. But either the union did not try or it was not able to generate nearly the same attention from the local paper or health officials about dangers inside the factory. Soon, new federal agencies such as the Environmental Protection Agency (EPA) as well as the Occupational Safety and Health Administration (OSHA) would be citing the Landrigan study, focused on children in the neighborhood, as providing some of the most conclusive evidence for reducing the lead allowed in the environment as well as workplaces, also in consumer goods such as gasoline. But only when OSHA itself began to intensify its scrutiny of conditions inside the smelter, during the late seventies, did reportage on these pick up some, even as measured lead levels in the air did decline significantly.[21]

Many of us have lived of professional lives through the changes that resulted from this kind of conflict, and this kind of science. The new environmental sciences, groups and movements have long since become familiar, along with the agencies and laws that, back then, provided hopeful new frameworks for struggles. The changes, from new kinds of epidemiology to the emergence of federal oversight, also had major impacts in the realm of occupational health in the US. In part because of these accomplishments, however, our own present looks a lot different from that of the 1970's. So much so that we may speak of it as a third phase in the twentieth to twenty-first century history of industrial hazards. Over the last decades, public attentiveness to hazards inside the workplace has stood even less of chance, as unions have been rapidly losing what share it had of the American workforce. Reasons for this decline are rooted not only in changes in politics but in the shrinking presence of factories on the American landscape. Most of our extraction, and not just the heavier but all aspect of production itself, now takes place abroad. So too, the most severe and dangerous of the workplace hazards, through which the commodities purchased by Americans are made. A recent depiction of how pollution happens, on the Environmental Protection Agency (EPA) website, captures this "post-industrial" detachment from the factory in an idealized form. In this cartoon, the polluting factories with which the agency is concerned have no people in or around them. They lie at some distance, and across a river, from a city where people are shown, as well as the rural places where they are show at play. [22]

Once again, the historical study of industrial localities, like this one in El Paso, illustrates what such an image gets right but also what it leaves out. By the mid-1970's, ASARCO and El Paso officials had effectively shut down Smeltertown, the most exposed community of Hispanic families right next to the smelter. By the mid 1980's it had closed its lead and zinc smelters, and in 1999 the final operation, a copper smelter, was shuttered. For all these retreats, however, the mobilizations against ASARCO continued to build. From the 1980's, many of these followed in the mold of what became known as an Environmental Justice Movement. Their concern was with all the lead and other contaminants left in the soil, even as the plant itself was shutting down. This is a movement that continued to gather steam into the 2000's.[23] But by this time, it was confronting a company that was no longer American owned; Grupo Mexico had bought ASARCO out. And the site of lead production itself had also shifted decisively. Fifty years before the El Paso smelter had been among the hemisphere's largest. By the 1990's, that reputation was now overtaken by smelters in Torreon, Mexico, and Peru, far south of the American border.[24]

These circumstances have brought a third phase in the kind of media attention to industrial hazards in the United States, suggested in this slide. After peaking around 1970, the fascination with industrial pollution has arguably undergone a slide similar to changes in coverage of occupational hazards over prior decades. With the EPA in charge, with experts increasingly empowered and clean air and water acts being implemented, also with the endless quest of the media itself for news-worthy novelties, coverage of pollution itself, as connected with industry, also gradually slide. The slide did not prove as thorough-going as that of workplace dangers. But it was real nonetheless. And with the exception of a punctuation mark in the late eighties, thanks to Bhopal and Chernobyl, along with the Exxon Valdez, it has been accompanied by declining concern about pollution in nationwide polls.

The good news here, at least in terms of public attention to the kinds of dangers that concern us, is that another kind of media coverage of hazards has proven more sustainable. That is reflected in the usage of "toxic" or "toxin" here. Talk about the toxic had roots in the early twentieth century American workplace; you'll recall that Alice Hamilton titled her first textbook for the budding field as "industrial toxicology."[25] But newspapers largely shied away from this usage until the explosion of environmental science and regulation during the 1970's. And while the early adopters were largely concerned with "toxic" wastes from industry, the usage itself has taken stable root in our public discourse largely through talk about consumer exposures. Now granted, this kind of concern goes back much further; to find earlier versions of it you need only trace the early history of the FDA. What's interesting, however, is how it has emerged over the last while as a kind of popular bridging terminology, for all those types of dangers to which our still de-industrializing society remains exposed. Its applications are widespread, from the leaded toys discovered on our department store shelves, to the Toxic America, recently portrayed on a CNN special.[26]

It will be interesting to see how the Gulf Oil spill's impact plays out on these fronts, whether it betokens a reversal of these long-term trends, though the historical record does not suggest a transformative change can come from any single disaster. Among the consequences I would like to draw for us today, a wide range of topics beckon for study in the history of occupational and environmental health, besides a kind of self-congratulatory history of our fore-bearers. On the one hand, I think it is important to devise our own ways of resisting the tides of media coverage and prioritizing. My evidence suggests that occupational hazards are arguably the biggest blindspot of American reporters today, yet we need more scrutiny of just how and why this may have happened. We also need much more attention to historical questions to where and how industrial hazards themselves have been moving, and what the consequences have been. But by the same token, I think we can draw a conclusion that these shifts in media coverage indicate just how much more extensive, over the past century, the sway of the US's industrial hazard regime has at least officially become. It now includes exposures inside the workplace, those outside, and also those wastes that have persisted, even long after the factories that produced them have vanished or migrated.

These days, as I have sought to suggest, we can also learn much by, instead of merely celebrating our fore-bearers, also asking questions about what they didn't see. This means reconstructing histories not just of heroic practitioners, but of industrial localities, like this region of El Paso. It also means applying a more searching scrutiny of our expert fore-bearers of a given era. By attending not just to hazards they recognized and acted upon but those that they did not, we will be composing a history that is not so exclusively congratulatory, that is also critical. Precisely such an orientation to the past, I wish to suggest, can better prepare today's experts to be more open and receiving of history-making changes in their own future.

Notes

[1] Campbell Robertson, '11 Remain Missing After Oil Rig Explodes Off Louisiana', *New York Times*, 22 April 2010, p. A23; Ian Urbina and Justin Gillis, 'Workers on Oil Rig Recall Terrible Night of Blast', *New York Times*, 8 May 2010, p. 1A; Faucet, 'Oil Rig Explodes; 11 Missing', *Los Angeles Times*, 22 April 2010, p. 1A; Richard Faucet, 'Oil Spill Far Bigger Than Thought', *Los Angeles Times*, 29 April 2010, p. 1A; 'Chicago Firm Helping BP with Tide of Spill Suits', *Chicago Tribune*, 18 May 2010; 'Gulf of Mexico Spill Reaches Louisiana Coast', *Washington Post*, 30 April 2010, p. 1A.

[2] Alice Hamilton, *Exploring the Dangerous Trades: The Autobiography of Alice Hamilton, M.D.* (Boston, Mass.: Northeastern University Press, 1985); Christopher Sellers, 'Factory as Environment: Industrial Hygiene, Professional Collaboration and the Modern Sciences of Pollution', *Environmental History Review*, 18 (1994), 55ff.

[3] The notion was first suggested in the concluding discussion at a 2007 conference held Stony Brook University. The definition we have developed of it loosely parallels that of the "urban regime" which has helped enable comparative study of cities: Clarence Stone, *Regime Politics: Governing Atlanta, 1946-88* (Lawrence, KA: University of Kansas Press, 1989), 6; Karen Mossberger and Gerry Stoker, "The Evolution of Urban Regime Theory; the Challenge of Conceptualization," *Urban Affairs Review* 36(2001):810-35. It also builds on Murphy's notion of "regimes of imperceptibility," Michelle Murphy, 'Chemical Regimes of Living', *Environmental History*, 13 (2008), 695-703; *Dangerous Trade: Histories of Industrial Hazard Across a Globalizing World*, ed. by Christopher Sellers and Joseph Melling (Philadelphia: Temple University Press, 2011).

[4] Franz Koelsch, *Bernardino Ramazzini - Der Vater Der Gewerbehygiene, 1633-1714* (Stuttgart: F. Enke, 1912); Henry E. Sigerist, 'Historical Background of Industrial and Occupational Diseases', *Bulletin of the New York Academy of Medicine*, 12 (1936), 597-609; L.J. Goldwater, 'From Hippocrates to Ramazzini: Early History of Industrial Medicine', *Ann. Medical History*, 8 (1936), 27-35.

[5] Bernardino Ramazzini, *A Treatise of the Diseases of Tradesmen Shewing the Various Influence of Particular Trades Upon the State of Health, with the Best Methods to Avoid or Correct It, and Useful Hints Proper to Be Minded in Regulating the Cure of All Diseases Incident to Tradesmen* (London: Printed for Andrew Bell [and 8 others], 1705); Koelsch; G E Hook, 'Ramazzini: Father of Environmental Health?', *Environmental Health Perspectives*, 103 (1995), 982-983.

[6] Rainer Müller, *Beiträge Zur Geschichte Der Arbeiterkrankheiten Und Der Arbeitsmedizin in Deutschland, Schriftenreihe Der Bundesanstalt Für Arbeitsschutz. Sonderschrift*; S 15; Variation: Sonderschrift (Bundesanstalt Für Arbeitsschutz (Germany)); 15. (Dortmund: Bundesanstalt für Arbeitsschutz, 1984); P. W. J. (Peter W. J.) Bartrip, *The Home Office and the Dangerous Trades: Regulating Occupational Disease in Victorian and Edwardian Britain*, Wellcome Series in the History of Medicine; Clio Medica; 68; Variation: Wellcome Series in the History of Medicine; Clio Medica (Amsterdam, Netherlands); 68. (Amsterdam; New York: Rodopi, 2002); Carolyn Malone and Royal Historical Society (Great Britain), *Women's Bodies and Dangerous Trades in England, 1880-1914* (Woodbridge, Suffolk, New York: Boydell Press, 2003); Christopher C Sellers, *Hazards of the Job: From Industrial Disease to Environmental Health Science* (Chapel Hill: University of North Carolina Press, 1997).

[7] Much of this and subsequent discussion draws on Sellers; also Christopher Sellers, 'A Prejudice That May Cloud the Mentality: The Making of Modern Objectivity in American Industrial Medicine,' in *Silent Victories; History and Progress of Public Health in America* (New York: Oxford University Press, 2006), pp. 230-52.

[8] Alice Hamilton, *Exploring the Dangerous Trades; the Autobiography of Alice Hamilton, M. D.* (Boston, Little, Brown and company, 1943); Alice Hamilton, U. S. Department of Labor and Bureau of Labor Statistics, Industrial Poisons Used or Produced in the Manufacture of Explosives, Bulletin of the United States Bureau of Labor Statistics; No. 219; Industrial Accidents and Hygiene Series; No. 14; Bulletin of the United States Bureau of Labor Statistics; No. 219; Bulletin of the United States Bureau of Labor Statistics; Industrial Accidents and Hygiene Series; Variation: Bulletin of the United States Bureau of Labor Statistics; No. 219; Bulletin of the United States Bureau of Labor Statistics; Industrial Accidents and Hygiene Series. (Washington: Government Printing Office, 1913); Allan McLaughlin, 'International Boundary Water Commission's Investigation of Sewage Pollution

of Boundary Waters', American Journal of Public Health, 5 (1915), 555-59.

[9] Wellington Donaldson, 'Industrial Wastes in Relation to Water Supplies', *American Journal of Public Health*, 11 (1921), 193-98; Frederick William. Fisher Lane and others, Effect of Oil Pollution of Coast and Other Waters on the Public Health, Bauer, Arthur D., Variation: Public Health Reports; V. 39, No. 28, July 11, 1924 (p. 1657-1662) (Washington, Govt. Print. Off., 1924); David Stradling, *Smokestacks and Progressives: Environmentalists, Engineers, and Air Quality in America, 1881--1951* (The Johns Hopkins University Press, 2002).

[10] 'Sewage Killing Off Fish in the Harbor', New York Times, 12 July 1908, p. 5; also 'Must Clean Waters Around New York', *New York Times*, 20 September 1912, p. 8.

[11] Hamilton; Alice Hamilton, Lead Poisoning in the Smelting and Refining of Lead, *Bulletin of the United States Bureau of Labor Statistics* (Washington: G.P.O., 1914), CXLI; United States. Division of Labor Standards, Occupational Disease Coverage in the Compensation Acts of U.S., Canada, England (Washington. Government Printing Office, 1936); David Edmondson and others, 'History of ASARCO in El Paso' (Office of Senator Eliot Shapleigh, 2007).

[12] Anita Chan and Robert J. S. Ross, 'Racing to the Bottom: International Trade Without a Social Clause', Third World Quarterly, 24 (2003), 1011-1028; Jackie Simpkins, 'The Global Workplace: Challenging the Race to the Bottom', Development in Practice, 14 (2004), 110-118; Aseem Prakash and Matthew Potoski, 'Racing to the Bottom? Trade, Environmental Governance, and ISO 14001', *American Journal of Political Science*, 50 (2006), 350-364.

[13] Among these studies are those of the environs of the El Paso smelter itself: P J Landrigan and others, 'Epidemic Lead Absorption Near an Ore Smelter. The Role of Particulate Lead', *New England Journal of Medicine*, 292 (1975), 123-9 <doi:1196336>; B Raquel Ordóñez, L Ruiz Romero and I R Mora, '[Epidemiological Study of Lead Levels in the Child Population and the Household Environment in Ciudad Juárez, Chihuahua, Mexico, as Compared to a Foundry Area in El Paso, Texas]', Boletín De La Oficina Sanitaria Panamericana, 80 (1976), 303-17 <doi:130912>.

[14] 'Forty Years Ago', *El Paso Herald-Post*, 17 March 1937, p. 4; 'Smoke from Smelter Gives Profit', *El Paso Herald-Post*, 19 May 1938, p. 12; '20.000 Tons of Invisible Gas Issue Daily from Smelter Stack', *El Paso Herald-Post*, 15 July 1937, p. 10.

[15] Hazel Erskine, 'The Polls: Pollution and Its Costs', *The Public Opinion Quarterly*, 36 (1972), 120-135.
[16] 'New Compensation Insurance Rates to Apply Sept. 5', *Brownsville Herald*, 7 August 1947, p. 9.
[17] John Abersold and K.W. Nelson, 'Industrial Hygiene at American Smelting and Refining Company', *Transactions of the American Institute of Mining and Metallurgical Engineers*, 191 (1951), 33-36.
[18] 'State Officials Study El Paso Smog Problem', *El Paso Herald-Post*, 6 February 1953, p. 1.
[19] Christopher Sellers, *Unsettling Ground: Suburban Nature and the Rise of Environmentalism in Twentieth-Century America* (Chapel Hill: University of North Carolina Press, 2012).
[20] Edmondson and others; Landrigan and others, 123-9.
[21] 'ASARCO Controls Demanded', *El Paso Herald-Post*, 26 February 1972, p. 1 (quote); on levels in 1975, also on late seventies/early eighties decline, see 'Letter of John R. Pritchard Regarding the Use of Respirators in ASARCO Plants, Docket OSHA-H033C-2006-0917-1174' (OSHA, 1984) <http://www.regulations.gov/#!searchResults;rpp=10;so=DESC;sb=postedDate;po=0;s=OSHA-H033C-2006-0917-1174> [accessed 14 February 2011].
[22] Image from 2004 accessed 2/2010 at http://www.epa.gov/indicate/roe/pdf/EPA_Draft_ROE.pdf
[23] Monica Perales and William P. Clements Center for Southwest Studies, *Smeltertown: Making and Remembering a Southwest Border Community* (Chapel Hill: University of North Carolina Press, 2010); Edmondson and others; Christian Warren, *Brush with Death: A Social History of Lead Poisoning* (Baltimore, MD: Johns Hopkins University Press, 2000); Peter C English, *Old Paint: A Medical History of Childhood Lead-Paint Poisoning in the United States to 1980* (New Brunswick, NJ: Rutgers University Press, 2001); Gerald E Markowitz and David Rosner, *Deceit and Denial: The Deadly Politics of Industrial Pollution* (Berkeley, CA: University of California Press, 2002).
[24] CDC, "Blood Lead Levels and Risk Factors for Lead Poisoning Among Children in Torreón, Coahuila, Mexico" (1998) accessed 2/11/2011 at http://www.bvsde.paho.org/bvsea/fulltext/torreon.pdf.
[25] Alice Hamilton, *Industrial Toxicology*, (New York, Harper, 1934).
[26] "Toxic America" accessed 2/11/2011 at: http://www.cnn.com/SPECIALS/2010/toxic.america/

Comment

Occupation, Environment and Health:
A History of Interdependence

Dan Berman, Ph.D.
Independent Scholar, Davis, CA, USA

It is one thing to isolate a deadly microbe but quite another to identify, by name, a life-threatening place of employment or clearly pinpoint a hazardous environmental epicenter. Ibsen understood this in *An Enemy of the People*, his play describing the ostracism of a medical doctor after he threatens the local tourist-based economy by revealing pollution of the town's bathing spring...by industrial tannery waste."

Paul D. Blanc, *How Everyday Products Make People Sick*[1]

In his presentation, Sellers defined industrial hazard regimes" as "social arrangements, formal as well as informal, by which public bodies, private interests, and civic mobilizations handle the danger and damage associated with an industry" each "with its own versions of novelty and spectacle." Sellers argued that during the 20th century there had been "an apparent evolution of spatial priorities" in which "industrial hazards outside the workplace" have come to be portrayed as "far more spectacular and troubling than those to workers within."

After listing the barriers to solving pollution problems, Professor Sellers stated that over the last century there has been a shift in social attention from

1) "a narrower, workplace-centered notion" (1900 through the early 1920s) to

2) "industrial pollution" near factories (1925 through late 1960s) to a concept of

3) "pollution...detached from sites of production altogether" (late 1960s to the present).

He backed up this argument by noting how quickly the television news stopped covering the 11 workers killed in the BP oil well blowout in the Gulf this spring,[2] and quickly re-focused on the damage to seabirds, fish, plankton, coral, and seacoast marshes.

Sellers based much of his analysis on passages from Dr. Alice Hamilton's 1943 memoir *Exploring the Dangerous Trades*[3] and on El Paso newspaper coverage of the local ASARCO lead and zinc smelter over the decades until its closure in the 1980s. (Other media such as movie newsreels and radio, which became important in the 1930s, and TV, which became predominant to mass audiences in 1950s—are not discussed).

To illustrate his discussion of factory exposures, Sellers referred to Hamilton's description of conditions in 1916 *outside* a New Jersey munitions plant which was supplying high explosives to France. Here Hamilton wrote about the spectacular and even gruesomely comic aspect of the "canaries"—the workers whose hair and fingernails had been stained bright orange and yellow while working with picric acid. She also described herself "choking and gasping before the angry fumes...pouring over the spot where I stood" as well as "the lowlands blackened and festering in the sunlight" which turned the streams "into something poisonous." outside the plant. But none of those hellish extra-plant conditions—recalled in her memoir a quarter-century later—were of interest to the Department of Labor, which had tasked Hamilton to investigate conditions *within* the munition plants. I question whether the differences between evolving "hazard regimes" over the 20th century are as clear-cut as Dr. Sellers claims, especially the distinction between work-based and general environmental hazards.

In *Death On the Job*[4] what I called the "compensation-safety apparatus" might qualify as an "industrial hazard regime" in Sellers' terminology. The "compensation-safety apparatus"—a regime of mandatory workmen's compensation systems monopolized by private insurance firms and incompetent, state-administered industrial inspection systems—was adapted as a model by the National Civic Federation (NCF) from British and German precedents. The National Civic Federation was a coalition founded and funded by large corporations and a few unions were encouraged to join to make the group look even-handed. The identification of three distinct "industrial hazard regimes," based on the treatment of industrial pollution in the press, seems to miss the mark given that for workers throughout most of the 20th century there has existed only one "industrial hazard regime," a compensation-safety apparatus which slights their needs and has changed little over the over the decades.

By 1900, exposés of the horrors of the primitive working conditions in

America were old hat in what came to be called the "muckraking" mass-circulation weeklies like *Everybody's* and *McClure's Magazine.* And Socialist Party magazines like the weekly Appeal to Reason, with press runs of 500,000 to 750,000 in the first decade and a half of its existence, also published a great deal about the issues of job health and safety. Indeed, the *Appeal* helped fund *The Jungle*, a 1906 novel by Upton Sinclair that highlighted the dangerous and filthy conditions faced by immigrant workers in the Chicago stockyards which became an instant best-seller.

By the time foundation-sponsored books such as Crystal Eastman's *Work-Accidents and the Law* (1910) and John Fitch's *The Steel Workers* (1911) appeared, big business and the insurance companies had already come up with their preferred solution to job safety problems, operating closely through business-dominated groups like the National Civic Federation. The NCF "solution"—sketched in the Eastman book—was a workmen's compensation[5] system which became the sole legally actionable remedy in cases of industrial injury or death. The system of special workmen's compensation referees and judges which was created in this system set low caps on benefits, especially for very costly permanent disability cases, so that payouts would be small and predictable, while the newly-installed state-level workmen's compensation system forbade workers from taking their grievances to civil or criminal court for trial by jury. By 1920, the NCF model had "solved" the problem of industrial safety at a cost to employers of only 1% of payroll on the average. There was only minimal interference from weak state-based industrial inspection systems, manned predominantly by ill-trained, low-paid political appointees. The fines and punishments levied against employers constituted mere slaps on the wrist, if invoked at all. For example, in Missouri, from 1925 through 1969, all industrial inspectors were political appointees who lost their jobs whenever the governorship changed hands from Republican to Democratic or vice-versa.[6] The newly installed workers' compensation systems made it nearly impossible to win compensation for permanently disabling injuries or occupational diseases.

The new compensation-safety apparatus, under the guise of reform, constituted a win for most employers, because costs were low and predictable, jury trials for work accidents were outlawed, and business owners no longer had to worry that the issue of working conditions could be used to challenge the legitimacy of corporate rule. What had been the "bloody bright issue of industrial slaughter" had been transformed into a dull-as-dishwater series of interminable bureaucratic tugs-of-war between injured workers and their former employers which had the net effect of keeping this vital issue off the front pages. It was great victory for the owners of industry.

Since the blossoming of the "new" environmental movement in the 1960s and 1970s, the corporate interests have been trying to replicate thet cost-saving victory of workers compensation, as citizens became more aware of general environmental problems. Since the public at large can take its grievances to courts for trial before juries of their peers, an aroused public has had greater success than the workers' movement in campaigning for bans on dangerous substances and in securing more stringent regulatory remedies. Certainly, as Sellers argues, there have always been complementary interactions between the workplace and environment at large, and, over the years, the relative importance of public attention to extra-workplace threats—highlighted by occasional multi-million-dollar judgments against corporate polluters—has come to overshadow in-plant safety problems. But this is hardly a novel idea for those who recall Upton Sinclair's famous quip regarding *The Jungle*: "I aimed for the heart and hit the stomach."

By the mid-1920s, the interaction between the occupational and the general environmental issues over the strongly contested issue of the production and use of tetraethyl lead (TEL) as a gasoline additive—as laid out in the writings of historians Gerald Markowitz and David Rosner—could not be clearer.[7] Dozens of workers were killed and many scores more were seriously poisoned at General Motors, Du Pont, and Standard of New Jersey during the production and blending of TEL into gasoline, which was introduced in order to raise octane level and thus the power and speed of gasoline engines.

Alice Hamilton of Harvard, and Yandell Henderson of Yale, as well as Grace Burnham of the pioneering (but short-lived) Workers Health Bureau strongly protested the introduction of highly toxic tetraethyl lead (TEL) as a gasoline additive in 1924-25, soon after its market launch. Their protest was based on its lethal effects on workers and as well as its likely damage to the population at large.

"You may control conditions within the factory," wrote Hamilton, "but how are you going to control the whole country?" Henderson called the new additive "one of the most dangerous things in the country" and correctly predicted that problems with its use would grow "insidiously" over the years. Grace Burnham, drawing on estimates from Standard of New Jersey, predicted that the 15 million gallons a year in projected sales of leaded gasoline could be expected to spew 50,000 tons of lead onto the nation's highways and streets—a figure which quadrupled in fact to 190,000 tons a year by

1970[8]—exposing almost everybody in the United States to environmental lead pollution, especially those who lived near freeways and other busy thoroughfares. As a result of the scientific and frightened popular protest over TEL, Standard temporarily stopped sales of the additive, and New York City actually banned its sale for three years in the 1920s. Thus as early as the 1920s, the history of TEL could be seen as an "industrial hazard regime" localized regionally but with "pollution...detached from sites of production altogether," preceding by forty years the cases highlighted in books such as Rachel Carson's *Silent Spring* (1962), Gene Marine's *America the Raped* (1969) or Barry Commoner's *Science and Survival* (1971).

In the 1930s the issue of silicosis—which Markowitz and Rosner chronicle in meticulous detail in *Deadly Dust*[9]—was handily neutralized by the Air Hygiene Foundation, a new research and lobbying entity called into existence by Pittsburgh's Mellon Foundation. It was founded in response to an *ad hoc* coalition composed of labor unions plus a now progressive Department of Labor that sponsored a national conference on silicosis in April 1936 and whose nominal goal was to tighten up state-level compensation laws and beef up state-controlled industrial inspection capabilities. The Air Hygiene Foundation—reprising the role of the National Civic Federation 20 years earlier—took the lead in the defense of corporate prerogatives and dominated the silicosis conference. This turned out to be prelude to Air Hygiene's later success in minimizing the compensability of silicosis and other disabling lung diseases by marshalling the testimony of employer-friendly physicians in legislative/regulatory hearings and compensation cases. The result, nation-wide in the U.S., was to make sure that almost no compensation for permanent disability from dust diseases made it through the various state compensation systems: neither in West Virginia (where the Hawk's Nest tunnel had been drilled), nor in New York State, nor in the tri-state region of Oklahoma, Arkansas, and Missouri, where dozens of small silicosis-producing lead and zinc mines were located.

A second Department of Labor conference in 1940 on silicosis in the tri-state region resulted in little or no permanent aid for the miners who worked in thick clouds of sand-laden dust and often died of slow suffocation from silicosis, despite vigorous preventive campaigns by the International Union of Mine, Mill and Smelter Workers. After World War II, many of the tri-state mines shut down and miners who were still healthy found other jobs. At the same time the left-leaning Mine, Mill and Smelter Workers union, often led by Communists, was driven out of existence by organized Red-baiting and through the legal strictures of the Taft-Hartley and the Smith Acts. Indeed, no significant action regarding the prevention of dust diseases would happen until the passage of the Coal Mine Health and Safety of 1969 and the Occupational Safety and Health Act of 1970.

The ties between the modern struggles for safer workplaces and for a cleaner environment at large were reflected in the half-ironic title of Franklin Wallick's book *The American Worker: An Endangered Species* (1972). Wallick's book—now almost forgotten—highlighted on the contrasting statistics of 4,690 state fish and game wardens in U.S. at a time (1968, pre-OSHA) when there were only 1,204 state work safety inspectors, even generously lumping together all factory, elevator, boiler, and mine safety inspectors. Oklahoma was the most backward of the jurisdictions, with 30 times as many fish and game wardens as work safety inspectors (150 vs. 5); only in Connecticut and New York did the number of work safety inspectors exceed the number of game wardens.[10]

Among examples of successful worker safety initiatives, Wallick's book told the story of a model project at Teamsters Local 688 at the Crane Corporation in St. Louis, an effort in which I had personal experience. We successfully tested an investigative system called *A Job Health and Safety Program on a Limited Budget*, in which a group of unionized workers (led by shop steward Art Button and me) began to clean up a hot, smoky, steel pipe factory where giant half-cylinders of steel were welded together on two longitudinal seams.[11]

With the great Earth Day mobilization of millions in the spring of 1970, and the passage of the Environmental Policy Act, the OSHA Act, the Clean Water Act, and the Clean Air Act under President Nixon in 1970 and 1971, a new environmental movement began to assume national significance as a political force. Perhaps the fact that most of those laws dealt the general environment rather than the workplace per se exemplifies the interrelationship between the workplace (where the problems start) and the rest of the world where people and other beings live—between the great public outdoors and the great private indoors. Later on *The Song of the Canary*, a 1979 documentary film by Josh Hanig and David Davis, showed how in-plant dangers could spread to the environment at large. The film portrayed the shock of men as they figured out they were being sterilized at a pesticide plant where they worked. The Occidental Chemical plant in Lathrop, California produced DBCP, a pesticide which also sterilized thousands of agricultural workers when sprayed on bananas and other crops in Central and South

America and in the United States. *Song of the Canary* was a jolting illustration of the truism that "risks do not evaporate outside the factory door."[12]

Still, some diseases were so obviously the product of particular agents and conditions, that it was possible to organize mass campaigns to institute a federal law to guarantee compensation of black lung disease among coal miners and to reduce exposure to the coal dust which had caused it. In fact, the Black Lung Associations which were formed to campaign for black lung, as coal workers' pneumoconiosis came to be called, ended up forming the shock troops in a successful campaign to reform the United Mine Workers and remove its entrenched leadership that had pretended that black lung was not a significant problem for coal miners.[13]

In the case of asbestos, victims' attorneys found they could win lawsuits against asbestos *suppliers* through jury trials, avoiding the workers' compensation system altogether. By avoiding the tight damage ceilings for permanent disability under workers' compensation law, an estimated $100 billion has been paid out over the last 40 years in asbestos claims.[14] These large settlements, inconceivable under workers' comp, have led to a de facto ban on asbestos use in the United States. For decades the corporate sector has struggled—with some success—to limit or abolish third-party liability suits with their jury trials and occasional multi-million-dollar judgments. "We don't want this to turn into another asbestos" is the refrain of corporate executives and legal departments when challenged by accusations that one of their products may be a health threat to the general public.

To this day, the corporate interests motivated by profit continue to limit efforts to control to workplace and environmental hazards. Relative corporate influence over OSHA, for example, has increased dramatically in the last 35 years, as union membership has dwindled from 25% to 12% of the workforce ...with only 7% union membership in the private sector.

Freedom from unhealthy environments at work and in the world at large should be understood as basic public rights which are dependent on the organized social power of ordinary citizens. As such, healthy conditions on the job or in the broader environment are social conquests—like public schools and streets, police and fire-fighting services, and parks and playgrounds open to all citizens.

As many people know, the right to a safe working conditions and a clean environment have been under constant attack by business interests who claim they are "useless paperwork" or "too costly." The original intent of OSHA was to establish nationally enforceable standards which would ensure that workplaces were "free from recognizable hazards." The fact that half of OSHA and almost all workers' compensation programs are administered by the states means businesses can play states against each other in a "race to the bottom."[15] To trim worker protections and benefits. Strict enforcement of OSHA or proposed increases in workers' comp. benefits inevitably triggers business threats to shut down or leave for states or countries "with a better business climate." Analogous pressures operate against tighter OSHA standards at the national level. Business-friendly administrations like the recent one of George W. Bush know the drill: from 2001 through 2007 during his terms in office, OSHA officials issued 86% fewer "economically significant" regulations than were issued during a comparable period under President Clinton, according to the *Wall Street Journal*.[16] In the waning days of the Clinton administration, OSHA had passed a comprehensive ergonomics standard which could have covered millions of workers in hundreds of thousands of workplaces. But the Republican-controlled Congress repealed that initiative shortly after taking office in 2001, to great applause from the U.S. Chamber of Commerce and the National Association of Manufacturers. The ergonomics standard has yet to be reinstated under President Obama.

Corporations and their allies over the last century have perfected their techniques for delaying and questioning the need for stricter environmental standards, as David Michaels pointed out in *Doubt Is Their Product: How Industry's Assault on Science Threatens Your Health*.[17] As the Assistant Secretary of Labor for Occupational Safety and Health in the Obama administration, Dr. Michaels must now contend with a Republican majority in the House that began in January 2011. Clearly he has his work cut out for him.

NOTES

[1] *How Everyday Products Make People Sick: Toxins At Home and in the Workplace*, Berkeley, University of California Press, 2007, p. 2. Blanc's elegantly written book follows the history and risks of dozens products and their hazards fronn glue to gasoline.

[2] The well blew out on April 20, 2010 and was finally capped in late summer 2010.

[3] Boston, Little Brown and Company, 1943.

[4] Daniel M. Berman, *Death On the Job: Occupational Health and Safety Struggles in the United States,* New York, Monthly Review Press, 1978,

esp. ch. 4, "The Compensation-Safety Apparatus." Chapter 1, "Why Work Kills," sketches the origin of the *apparatus*, and a few of its typical *apparatchiki* make appearance throughout the book.

[5] Called "workers' compensation" since around 1968 as the women's movement gained traction.

[6] Cited in Berman, *Death On the Job*, op. cit., p. 56.

[7] Gerald Markowitz and David Rosner, "A 'Gift of God': The Public Health Controversy over Leaded Gasoline during the 1920s," in the *American Journal of Public Health*, vol. 75, No. 4, pp. 344-352; also by Markowitz and Rosner and, *Deceit and Denial: The Deadly Politics of Industrial Pollution,* University of California Press, Berkeley, California, 2002, esp. Chapter 1, "The House of the Butterflies: Lead Poisoning among Workers and Consumers," pp. 12-35. Sellers covered this issue in depth as well in his book. See also Martin Cherniack's taut account of the Gauley Bridge killings in *The Hawk's Nest Incident: America's Worst Industrial Disaster*, New Haven, Yale University Press, 1986.

[8] The figure for motor vehicle lead emissions for 1970 is from "Interview with Barry Commoner," *Scientific America*, June 23, 1997, (downloaded on Oct 10, 2010) from
http://www.scientificamerican.com/article.cfm?id=interview-with-barry-comm&page=3. Martin By 1994, after TEL had been banned, emission of lead from cars and trucks had diminished to only 1,600 tons/year, according to Commoner.

[9] David Rosner and Gerald Markowitz, *Deadly Dust: Silicosis and the On-Going Struggle to Protect Workers' Health*, Ann Arbor, University of Michigan Press, 2006,

[10] Wallick, Franklin, *The American Worker: An Endangered Species:* New York, Ballantine Book, 1972, esp. pp. 162, 163 and 173-175. Wallick's book was reissued in a revised edition as *Don't Let Youir Job Kill You*, Progressive Press, New York, 1984 and is available on the internet. The book by Jeanne Stellman and Susan Daum, *Work Is Dangerous To Your Health*, New York, Pantheon, 1973) also has an account of the project at Teamsters Local 688.

[11] The work at Local 688 led to the engagement of Berman to head the Occupational Project of the Medical Cmmittee for Human Rights, out of Chicago and San Francisco, from the years 1972-1975, where we helped organize labor/medical/legal Committees for Occupational Safety and Health or "COSH groups" in cities around the United States.

[12] See Paul D. Blanc, *How Everyday Products Make People Sick: Toxins at Home and in the Workplace*, University of California Press, Berkeley, 2007, p. 3.
[13] Berman, *Death on the Job*, op. cit., pp. 136-142; also Alan Derickson, *Black Lung: Anatomy of a Public Health Disaster*, Ithaca and London, Cornell University Press, 1998.
[14] This estimate is by Dr. Barry Castleman, author of *Asbestos: Medical and Legal Aspects* (5th edition), New York, Aspen Publishers, 2005, 894pp. Castleman made the estimate to me over the telephone in late 2010.
[15] The expression was used by Professor John F. Burton, former head of the National Commission on State Workers' Compensation Law, to describe the attack on workers' compensation benefits in the last generation. See Burton's testimony before the Subcommittee on Workplace Protections, Committee on Education and Labor, United States Congress, November 17, 2010.
[16] Sarah Rubenstein, "OSHA Backs Off Workplace Health Warnings Under Bush," *Wall Street Journal,* December 29, 2010, view at http://blogs.wsj.com/health/2008/12/29/osha-backed-off-workplace-health-warnings-under-bush/.
[17] Published by New York Oxford University Press, 2008. For a talk on the theme of corporate dominance of the political process, check out Bill Moyers at the First Howard Zinn Memorial Lecture at Boston University, October 29, 2010, downloadable at http://www.bu.edu/buniverse/view/?v=20ZaW9PO.

Comment

Conceptualizing Hazards

Christine Meisner Rosen
Associate Professor, Haas School of Business
Associate Director for Business and Economy, Berkeley Center for Green Chemistry
University of California, Berkeley, CA, USA

In this paper, Christopher Sellers presents us with three important, thought provoking, interpretive points about the history of the American response to and understanding of industrial pollution emissions. The first is that despite the fact that the impact of industrial toxins on human health is essentially the same whether exposure occurs inside factories or outside them, Americans have, since the late nineteenth century, cognitively divided them into two distinct, general conceptual and political categories, in effect, converting them into very different species of hazard. We've perceived the hazardous emissions occurring inside factories to be a threat that is limited to the health and wellbeing of workers on the line—and as such, as an industrial hygiene problem that it is the responsibility of workers and their unions to fight and deal with through contract negotiations and state level occupational safety and health compensation and regulation.

Meanwhile, we've perceived the emissions occurring on the other side of the factory wall as a much bigger problem—as a threat to general public health, and, increasingly, to all living things, not to mention the climate as well as the physical beauty of the earth, problems against which environmental groups must organize to fight and governments regulate through zoning, pollution, and other environmental regulation. We frame these hazards as "environmental problems." They include our fears about the hazardous effects of the pollution streaming out of factory smokestacks and effluent pipes and worries about toxic contaminants in food, toys, furniture, and other consumer products, as well as our more abstract concerns about climate change, habitat destruction, and the destruction of natural resources.

Sellers' second point concerns the historical development of these conceptual categories. He argues that that Americans have not, for the most part, held these fears in our heads—or in our culture or our regulatory structures—simultaneously over time. Instead we have progressed through a sequential; three stage evolutionary process of recognizing, analyzing, and trying to deal with the different aspects of industrial pollution. From the late nineteenth century through the mid twentieth century, the narrower, work place centered notion prevailed and produced a regulatory regime that focused on the contractual protections and factory regulations. Starting in the late 1960s and early 1970s, around the time of the first Earth Day, a new set of fears came to the fore—one that obsessed over the harmful impacts of factory pollution on towns and cities. This produced a new regulatory regime that focused on end of pipe factory air and water pollution regulation. More recently, Sellers argues, we have lost interest in factory pollution and become obsessed with the toxins in consumer goods and the more general, abstract global environmental impacts of industrial activity—problems that he says are conceptually "detached from sites of production altogether." While he tells us that this staged process of development was more one of "layering on" than moving from a one set of ideas and a distinctive regulatory regime to new ones, in the paper he emphasizes the disjunctures between the phases. He argues that the earlier concerns disappeared from media accounts when new ones came to the fore, that the new fears produced novel regulatory industrial hazard regimes, and that the passage from one stage to the next led to a "characteristic patterns of oversight or neglect" of the old kind of hazard.

Sellers' third point is that this pattern has profoundly shaped the stories we historians write about the history of the American struggle with industrial toxins. We are as caught up in this step wise, disjunctive pattern as the rest of the American public. We have divided ourselves into separate specialties: historians of occupational safety and health who study the toxins in the workplace and environmental historians who study the history of urban and national struggles over factory and other industrial pollution; historians who study the 19th century, and others who study different eras in the 20th. As a result, we have not engaged with each other enough to recognize and investigate the general, longer term national historical pattern he's laying out for us here.

I wholeheartedly agree with much, but not all, of this. American ideas about industrial pollution have indeed evolved over time. I'm writing a book on the history of the American perception of and struggle with industrial pollution in the period between 1840 and the 1880s, from the perspective of environmental, business, urban, and legal history. The process by which new pollution beliefs emerged half way through this period is one of the primary focuses of the book. I also agree that Americans have a history of viewing view workplace toxic exposures and more general pollution problems as two separate problems—and that historians of occupational health and environmental historians have followed suit—and that we need to erase the lines that divide us and recognize how much we have in common, how interrelated our subject matters are, and how much we can learn from each other.

Sellers' three stage chronology is, however, in my view, much too simplistic. When I look at the history of society's response to industry's pollution emissions I see a longer and much more messy, complicated history. Decades before Alice Hamilton began investigating the diseases plaguing factory workers, Americans were deeply upset by and imposing regulations and legal sanctions on certain kinds of industrial environmental emissions, most notably the stenches emitted by slaughterhouses, rendering establishments, bone boiling concerns, soap and fertilizer factories. By the 1860s and 70s (a hundred years before anti-industrial pollution movements of the 1960s and 70s) outrage over the stenches emitted by manufactured gas plants and chemical and other factories not only led to lawsuits and regulatory efforts in New York City, but also a change in the case law in such heavily industrialized states as New York, Massachusetts, Pennsylvania, and New Jersey as judges began imposing injunctions and damages on the owners of the factories emitting foul smells, smokes, and water pollution. People still viewed the harmful effects of these noxious emissions through the lens of the miasmatic theory of disease, rather than modern toxicology science, but they nevertheless believed them to be threats to human health as well as human comfort and property values. During the 1890s and early 1900s, when Hamilton was hard at work studying and reporting on the diseases factory workers suffered, movements to regulate industrial and commercial smoke erupted in cities across the U.S. They led to scientific studies of the harmful effects of smoke on human health that resembled the occupational health studies conducted by Hamilton, most famously those published by Pittsburgh's Mellon Institute, as well as studies of the harmful economic costs of smoke and much work to develop and evaluate technologies for abating smoke pollution.

At the other end of Sellers' time continuum, in the 1960s, 70s, and 80s, work place health and environmental movements not only evolved simultaneously, they stimulated and reinforced each others' growth. News that asbestos workers brought asbestos diseases home to their families on their dusty work cloths and that the chemicals used to produce PVC were not only endangering factory workers, but also consumers, due to their presence in the aerosol propellants used in hairsprays, room deodorants, and spray paints fanned the public's fears, fuelling both union and environmentalist effort to achieve new protective regulations. It's true that in recent years, as more of American industrial production has moved abroad, the public has become increasingly interested in climate change, toxins in consumer goods, and other environmental problems, many with global rather than local dimensions, that have little to do with hazards in their local factories (if they have any). Yet it is also true that these broad new concerns engage unions and other kinds of worker groups in collaborative efforts, like the Apollo Alliance and the Blue Green Alliance, not only because growing numbers of American workers want the U.S. economy to produce more "green" jobs, but also because they see climate change and the toxins as threats to their own and the public's welfare.

The fact is that if the chronological stages in this history really were as separate and distinct as Sellers has argued—and if, as he suggests, the old understandings and concerns and regulatory regimes really had faded away after the new ones emerged—we environmental historians and historians of occupational safety and health would not have much in common, nor would we stand to benefit much from closer collaboration. But we do! Sellers is absolutely right when he argues we have much to learn from each other—because our histories are linked and interrelated in a myriad ways that need to be explored. I applaud Sellers' effort to inspire us to start working on integrating our histories and articulating analyses of how the different threads of the American struggle with industrial pollution have intersected and interacted over time. I also appreciate his effort to motivate us to probe the ways in which these threads have failed to intersect—despite the similarities and affinities between them. We need to examine all sides of the American struggle with industrial pollution.

Comment

Air Pollution and the Meuse Valley Fog of December 1930

Benoit Nemery, MD, PhD
Research Unit of Lung Toxicology
Department of Public Health
K.U.Leuven, Leuven, Belgium

THOSE WHO STUDY the adverse effects of air pollution often face problems with the very meaning and perception of the term "air pollution". For the general public—and, hence, the media and most politicians—air pollution is viewed essentially, if not solely, as the presence of unwanted pollutants in outdoor (or "ambient") air as a result of industrial or vehicular emissions, especially in urban areas. However, the air inside homes or in workplaces may also be polluted and, moreover, the concentrations of pollutants reached in indoor environments are often much higher than those reached outdoors.

Inside homes, air pollution is substantial when biomass—such as charcoal, wood, crop residues, or animal dung—is burnt for cooking and heating without adequate exhaust of the smoke. Thus, in poor countries, domestic exposure to biomass smoke may seriously affect the health of children and women, mainly in rural and mountainous areas.[1,2] The history of indoor pollution caused by cooking fires and its adverse effects on human health, from antiquity to modern times, is briefly sketched by Brimblecombe.[3]

Many people tend to disregard the occupational environment as belonging to the realm of air pollution, although the inhalation of pollutants at work is arguably responsible for more—and more severe—human disease than urban air pollution, even in modern industrialized countries. A well-known problem when studying the health effects of occupational exposures consists of the "healthy worker effect," a bias whereby working populations, especially in physically demanding jobs, are generally composed of healthy people, as a result of, first, selection of the fittest into the workforce and, later, exclusion from the workforce of those who become sick.[4] A lesser known (and hardly investigated) source of bias in occupational epidemiology is the "healthy workshop effect,"[5] which originates from the fact that good studies are more easily performed and more likely to be conducted in large companies—which are more likely to provide acceptable working conditions, as well as medical surveillance and, hence, medical records—than among non-organized workforces from small companies—who often have poor compliance with occupational hygiene regulations and no access to occupational medical services. This bias will tend to diminish the chances of demonstrating an adverse effect of work on health.

Similarly, tobacco smoking is not generally considered as a form of air pollution, yet this "do-it-yourself pollution" exposes the active smoker to quantities of irritant, toxic and carcinogenic gaseous agents and particulates that are far higher than in polluted urban environments. Consequently, cigarette smoking is undoubtedly a major and even the strongest risk factor for chronic respiratory and cardiovascular disease and cancer.[6] The relation between smoking and air pollution is relevant for the study of the history of the perception of the adverse health effects of occupational and environmental air pollution, because of two somewhat contradictory effects. On the one hand, urban air pollution and occupational exposures have been put forward to dismiss the possibility that smoking could cause lung cancer[7] and, later, specialists in occupational and environmental health have been "used" by the tobacco industry to divert attention from the risks of smoking.[8] Conversely, cigarette smoking has considerably complicated and obscured the discovery and documentation, as well as the management and compensation, of occupational and environmental health hazards. One important reason why the effects of smoking and occupation have been so difficult to disentangle from each other is that smoking and occupation are substantially confounded. Thus, at least in industrialized countries, the prevalence and intensity of smoking are generally higher among blue-collar workers than among white-collar workers and, among manual workers, those who have dirtier jobs are also more likely to be smokers.[9] In other words, "*the category of 'smoker' in a statistical sense is an index of likelihood of 'exposure' to occupational hazards.*"[10] Put another way, the fact that 80-90% of lung cancer is associated with smoking does not necessarily imply that only 10-20% are due to other causes. In practice, the overwhelming influence of smoking, has led many researchers and clinicians to ignore the role that dirty jobs play in the causation of respiratory diseases, such as chronic obstructive pulmonary disease

(COPD) or lung cancer. Similarly, poor communities and socially disadvantaged groups tend to be also more highly exposed (and more susceptible) to air pollution.[11,12]

Ambient air pollution

Links between urban air pollution and adverse health effects started to be made with the use of coal as a fuel in the seventeenth century.[3] This was particularly the case in London, as exemplified by John Evelyn's *Fumifugium, or the Smoake of London Dissipated* published in 1661. Interestingly, already in 1608, the authorities of Haarlem, Holland, banned the burning of coal within the city, because its inhabitants had expressed many complaints "*about the burning of English and Scottish coal ..., which produced over the whole city and in the houses of the citizens such a black dust, bad air and filthy matter of soot and ash that the linen, clothes and other goods became black and infected.*"[13] Ramazzini's *De Morbis Artificum Diatriba* (published in 1700) also contains the story of a citizen who complained of air pollution by sulphuric acid originating from a local workshop but, in this case, the judge ruled against the plaintiff.[14]

However, urban air pollution and its adverse effects on health became a matter of serious concern, with the industrial revolution, again mainly in London (3). The London fogs, which inspired artists such as Claude Monet (15), were both a sign of pollution and, when they became very dense, a cause of ill health. However, the first globally publicized and scientifically validated evidence that industrial pollution could kill did not come from London, but from a small area south of Liège in Belgium in 1930.[16,17]

The Meuse Valley fog of 1930

During the first week of December 1930, fog covered a large part of Europe, as a result of a severe temperature inversion. The fog was particularly intense along the valley of the Meuse river between the towns of Liège and Huy. This was a heavily industrialized area, where the industrial revolution had started in continental Europe. On the third day of the fog, i.e. on 3 December 1930, hundreds of people living in the villages along the Meuse started to suffer from respiratory troubles and at least 60 people died in respiratory distress over the course of the following three days, which represented a tenfold increase in mortality. Cattle was also affected. This event led to widespread coverage in the national and even international press, including the New York Times. That industrial pollution could be the cause of the disaster was not immediately recognized, and various other explanations for the mysterious "killer fog" were put forward in the media, such as the accidental release of chemical warfare agents—a few years earlier, during the first World War, the trenches of Ypres had been the theatre of the first large-scale use of chemical weapons—a recurrence of the Spanish flu—which had made millions of victims after the war—or an invasion by mysterious germs blown with a southerly wind coming from the Sahara. Not only was the lay press at a loss to explain the Meuse Valley disaster, also the medical and scientific world did not realize, at least initially, that industrial pollution could be the cause of the casualties. Thus, an anonymous piece in *The Lancet* of 13 December 1930, entitled "Fog panic on the Meuse," did not even evoke this possibility and simply discounted the hypothesis of any communicable disease as being responsible for the episode; the editorial did, however, point to the close association previously found by Mr. W.T. Russell between mortality and cold foggy weather.[18] However, soon thereafter it was accepted, according to an editorial in the British Medical Journal of 14 February 1931,[19] that "a continual stream of factory fumes [had been] prevented by the fog from escaping from the district; its concentration in the atmosphere steadily increased, therefore, and eventually, the limit of human tolerance was reached in some cases." The editorial concluded that "[f]or many years it has been urged that there is a need of a much stricter control over the smoke and fumes emerging from factory chimneys; the lesson of the deaths in the Meuse valley may conceivably have a wider application." This view seems to have largely resulted from the "closely argued report" by Prof. Storm van Leeuwen of Leyden, published on 9 January 1931 in the *Münchener medizinische Wochenschrift*.[20] Storm van Leeuwen "upon hearing the news that especially the asthmatics and bronchitics had become ill and died, [had driven] as quickly as possible to Liège", where he had a "great encounter" with Prof. Firket, the head of the multidisciplinary commission that had been charged by the royal prosecutor of Liège to investigate the "mechanisms of the accidents" that had led to the deaths.

The full report of the commission was produced within 6 months of the events and it was presented by Prof. Jean Firket to the Royal Academy of Medicine of Belgium on 19 May 1931.[16] The report was also published, in 1933, as part of a book on air pollution.[21] A shorter version of the report and its conclusions appeared in English, following a presentation by J. Firket to the Faraday Society in 1936.[22] As described in more detail elsewhere,[17] the report consisted of i/ a description of the symptoms, clinical features and autopsies in affected subjects; ii/ an analysis of the then prevailing meteorological conditions in the valley; iii/ an estimation of the toxic emissions by industry and domestic fires; and finally iv/ an interpretation of the most likely mechanisms to explain the observations. Patients mainly exhibited features of respiratory irritation and bronchial asthma; most of those who died were old and they generally had pre-existing pulmonary or cardiac disease. The weather was characterized by cold and intense fog, with low wind speed and a temperature inversion. The experts concluded that the most likely cause for the adverse health effects was the burning of coal by industry and domestic coal fires, thus resulting in high concentrations of SO_2 which could be transformed to sulphuric acid condensed on fine solid particles.

The investigation of the causes of Meuse Valley fog disaster represents a true landmark in the literature on air pollution. Even though its methods fell short of even the most basic epidemiological criteria, many conclusions that were reached by the authors are still valid now. Thus, the early identification of small particles as important contributors to the adverse health effects of air pollution is remarkable, because particulate matter (PM) is now generally accepted as the most hazardous component of urban air pollution. The experts also clearly concluded that the Meuse Valley disaster was not simply an act of God or a freak accident, but that the same accidents would occur in the valley or elsewhere, if the same circumstances were fulfilled. Prof. J.S. Haldane, one of the then leading respiratory physiologists in England, agreed more or less with these warnings, which were quite relevant in relation to the anticipated building of new power plants in London.[23]

In October 1948, a very similar deadly smog killed at least 20 people in Donora, a small industrial town with a large zinc smelter, south of Pittsburgh in Pennsylvania.[24] The Firket report calculated that a disaster like the one in the Meuse Valley would lead to more than 3000 deaths in London ["*Si un désastre survenait à Londres dans des conditions analogues on aurait à déplorer 3179 morts immédiates*"]. This happened during the infamous London smog of 5 to 9 December 1952, when between 3,000 and 4,000 people died.[25] Later research[26] would demonstrate that, in fact, many more people (approximately 12,000) died as a result of the pollution episode, since mortality remained higher than expected during many weeks after the fog had cleared.

Although the Meuse Valley disaster represents a true landmark in the history of industrial air pollution, very little has remained of this historical event in the affected area. At the end of the 20th century, the episode had all but disappeared from the collective memory among the people and the local authorities of Engis, where most deaths had occurred in 1930. However, on 2 December 2000 a statue was erected to the memory of the victims of this industrial catastrophe, thanks largely to the efforts of the late Valère Bovy – who had created a local committee for the protection of the environment ("*SOS Pays Mosan*") in 1972 after another (less deadly) air pollution incident.

Notes

[1] de Koning HW, Smith KR, Last JM. Biomass fuel combustion and health. *Bull World Health Organ* 1985;63(1):11-26.

[2] Smith KR, Sundell J. Human exposures to combustion products from household use of unprocessed solid fuels (biomass and coal) in simple stoves are substantial sources of ill-health in a world perspective. *Indoor Air* 2002 Sep;12(3):145-6.

[3] Brimblecombe P. Air pollution and health history. In: Holgate S, Samet JM, Koren HS, Maynard RL, editors. Air pollution and health.San Diego, London, Boston, New York, Sydney, Tokyo, Toronto: Academic Press; 1999. p. 5-18.

[4] Pearce N, Checkoway H, Kriebel D. Bias in occupational epidemiology studies. *Occup Environ Med* 2007 Aug;64(8):562-8.

[5] Nemery B, Casier P, Roosels D, Lahaye D, Demedts M. Survey of cobalt exposure and respiratory health in diamond polishers. *Am Rev Respir Dis* 1992;145:610-6.

[6] Ezzati M, Lopez AD. Estimates of global mortality attributable to smoking in 2000. *Lancet* 2003 Sep 13;362(9387):847-52.

[7] Clemmesen J. Lung cancer from smoking: delays and attitudes, 1912-1965. *Am J Ind Med* 1993;23:941-53.

[8] Diethelm PA, Rielle JC, McKee M. The whole truth and nothing but the truth? The research that Philip Morris did not want you to see. *Lancet* 2005 Jul 2;366(9479):86-92.

[9] McCurdy SA, Sunyer J, Zock JP, Anto JM, Kogevinas M. Smoking and occupation from the European Community Respiratory Health Survey. *Occup Environ Med* 2003 Sep;60(9):643-8.

[10] Sterling T, Weinkam J. The confounding of occupation and smoking and its consequences. *Soc Sci Med* 1990;4:457-67.

[11] O'Neill MS, Jerrett M, Kawachi I, Levy JI, Cohen AJ, Gouveia N, et al.

Health, wealth, and air pollution: advancing theory and methods. *Environ Health Perspect* 2003 Dec;111(16):1861-70.
[12] Wheeler BW, Ben-Shlomo Y. Environmental equity, air quality, socioeconomic status, and respiratory health: a linkage analysis of routine data from the Health Survey for England. *J Epidemiol Community Health* 2005 Nov;59(11):948-54.
[13] Biersteker K. Luchtverontreiniging in Haarlem in 1608 [Air pollution in Haarlem in 1608]. *Ned Tijdschr Geneeskd* 1968 Jan 6;112(1):33-4.
[14] Tedeschi CG. Bernardino Ramazzini (1633-1714): De Morbis Artificum. *Hum Pathol* 1970;1(2):315-9.
[15] Bates DV. A perspective on air pollution. *J Allergy Clin Immunol* 2005 Feb;115(2):432-4.
[16] Firket M. Sur les causes des accidents survenus dans la vallée de la Meuse, lors des brouillards de décembre 1930. Résultats de l'expertise judiciaire faite par MM. Dehalu, Schoofs, Mage, Batta, Bovy et Firket. *Bull Acad Roy Méd Belg* 1931;11:683-734.
[17] Nemery B, Hoet PH, Nemmar A. The Meuse Valley fog of 1930: an air pollution disaster. *Lancet* 2001 Mar 3;357(9257):704-8.
[18] Anonymous. Fog panic on the Meuse. *Lancet* 1930 Dec 13;ii:1305.
[19] Anonymous. Atmospheric pollution and pulmonary diseases. *Br Med J* 1931 Jan;1:277.
[20] Storm van Leeuwen W. Die Nebelkatastrophe im Industriegebiet südlich von Lüttich. *Münch.Med.Wochenschr.* 1931;78:49-50.
[21] Batta G, Firket J, Leclerc E. Les problèmes de pollution de l'atmosphère. Liège: Georges Thone; 1933.
[22] Firket J. Fog along the Meuse valley. *Transactions of the Faraday Society* 1936;32:1192-7.
[23] Haldane J. Atmospheric pollution and fogs. *Br Med J* 1931 Feb 28;1:366-7.
[24] Schrenk HH, Heimann H, Clayton GD, Gafafer WM, Wexler H. Air Pollution in Donora, PA: Epidemiology of the Unusual Smog Episode of October 1948, Preliminary Report. Public Health Bulletin No 306 Washington, DC:U S Public Health Service 1949.
[25] Wilkins ET. Air pollution and the London fog of December, 1952. *Journal of the Royal Sanitary Institute* 1954;74:1-21.
[26] Bell ML, Davis DL. Reassessment of the lethal London fog of 1952: novel indicators of acute and chronic consequences of acute exposure to air pollution. *Environmental Health Perspectives* 2001 Jun;109 Suppl 3:389-94.

Keynote

"An Injury to One is an Injury to All": Movements for Occupational and Environmental Health in Twentieth-Century America

Gerald Markowitz, PhD
University Distinguished Professor
John Jay College and CUNY Graduate Center
City University of New York

David Rosner, MSPH, PhD
Ronald H. Lauterstein Professor of Sociomedical Sciences and History
Columbia University and Mailman School of Public Health
New York, New York, USA

FOR MANY THE history of movements for occupational safety and health begins in the 1960s when union activists, particularly Tony Mazzocchi, the extraordinary leader of the Oil, Chrmical and Atomic Workers Union (OCAW), mobilized hundreds of thousands of workers and their unions to push for federal legislation that ultimately resulted in the passage of the Mine Safety and Health Act in 1969and the Occupational Safety and Health Act in 1970. These pieces of federal legislation resulted in the creation of the Mine Safety and Health Administration in the Department of the Interior, the Occupational Safety and Health Administration in the Department of Labor and the National Institute of Occupational Safety and Health in the National Institutes of Health. OSHA in particular was groundbreaking because it established for the first time the principle that workers had a right to a safe and healthful workplace and that the Federal government had a responsibility to ensure this through inspection, regulation and standard setting.

As Mazzocchi himself told OCAW members at a meeting in West Virginia near the site of the Gauley Bridge tunnel disaster of the early 1930s: "most of us probably never knew that 600 human beings perished building this particular aqueduct that would carry water to a plant where OCAW members are employed today."[1]

Certainly, the historiography of the past twenty five years has dramatically revised this narrative. The scholarship of people such as Dan Berman, Paul Blanc, Alan Derickson, Allison Helper, Jo Melling, Chris Sellers, Barbara Sicherman, Sarah Vogel and many others have added a level of depth and sophistication to the earlier historical account.[2] Yet, underlying Mazzocchi's analysis was a central truth: that until these historians and others began to reconstruct that history, the struggles to protect workers' health that were initiated by a movement of workers, reformers, and radicals were not a part of the official narrative of labor or social history. This was not because labor didn't "care" about health, but because the issue of occupational disease and disaster was folded in to the history of the broader struggle over working conditions, working class survival and other pressing social concerns.

Here we will look back at the first half of the 20th century. We will center on two periods—the first between 1900 and 1917, commonly known as the Progressive Era, and the second, the 1930s, the Depression and New Deal—to examine two different movements for addressing the horrendous conditions for workers in the United States. In the earlier period, labor, progressive reformers, radicals and socialists, social workers and others united to demand that the worst excesses of laissez faire capitalism be ameliorated and that the state protect workers' lives and health. In the New Deal era, the effort was less a movement than an uprising by workers discarded by industrial capitalism who used the courts to redress their individual harms, but in so doing changed popular and professional understanding of chronic industrial disease and initiated broad political and social changes.

The early movement built on existing state factory-inspection programs and efforts in the 1880s and 1890s to enact protective legislation for women and children. It reached its peak during the first two decades of the 20th century and garnered support among reformers working in public health, conservation, housing, and labor legislation. Contemporary discussion of occupational safety and health was wedded to broader social concerns regarding workers' housing, sanitation, and general living conditions. It was a "many-sided movement" where workers, social workers, housing reformers, journalists, politicians, big business representatives, social scientists, professionals, socialists, wobblies, and charity workers, who rarely agreed on much of anything, found themselves in alliance to stop the slaughter of workers in American industry. It brought together radical and conservative groups in sometimes tense coalitions.[3]

The growing concern over safety and health issues in the first decade of the 20th century arose in the wake of the revolutionary social and economic changes that America had just undergone. In little more than three decades Americans had witnessed the virtual explosion of urban and manufacturing centers. Between 1860 and 1890 the percentage of Americans living in cities tripled from a little more that 15 percent of Americans lived in cities by 1860 but by 1900 about 40 percent were urban. In terms of raw numbers the urban population increased seven fold between the end of the Civil War and 1905.

This was shocking to Americans reared in rural settings. Before the Civil War, most Americans lived on farms or in small towns; the few factories that existed were scattered in mill towns and villages in the Northeast. With the growth of the transcontinental railroads, however, the development of national markets, increased exploitation of natural resources such as coal and iron, and the massive immigration of labor from rural Europe to the cities of the East and Midwest, conditions of work changed dramatically. Speed-ups, monotonous tasks, exposure to chemical toxins, metallic and organic dusts, and unprotected machinery made the American workplace among the most dangerous in the world. In the United States more than 3 miners in every 1,000 could expect to die while working in a mine during any given year.[4]

Death, disability and disease were symptoms of the larger battles over unsafe and unhealthful working conditions, the eight hour day that were the focus of the various strikes and disruptions that marked the period. Generally, the issue of health was imbedded in broader struggles. But disease and death sometimes were the specific focus of labor disputes. Throughout the twentieth century health and work conditions were a staple concern in working class culture. Songs such as Union Miners began with descriptions of rocks falling and dangers of drilling. "Miner's life is like a sailors board a ship that crossed the waves; every day his life's in danger yet he stand up being brave; watch the rocks, they're falling daily, careless miners always fail," begins one song (http://www.youtube.com/watch?v=tJyioISLYHU). Another miners' ballad speaks to the dangers in the darkness: "Dark as a dungeon and damp as the dew where the dangers are many and the pleasures are few." http://www.youtube.com/watch?v=9s3_1OcFSHQ)

The enormous wealth produced by the new industrial plants was achieved at an inordinate social cost. "To unprecedented prosperity ... there is a seamy side of which little is said," responded one observer in 1907. "Thousands of wage earners, men, women and children, [are] caught in the machinery of our record breaking production and turned out cripples. Other thousands

[are] killed outright," he reported. "How many there [are] none can say exactly, for we [are] too busy making our record breaking production to count the dead."[5] In a theme that would repeatedly appear reformers compared the toll of industrial accidents to an undeclared war. As early as 1904 *The Outlook*, a mass-circulation magazine, commented on the horrendous social effects of industrialization. "A greater number of people are killed every year by so-called accidents than are killed in many wars of considerable magnitude," it pointed out. "It is becoming as perilous to live in the United States as to participate in actual warfare."[6]

The power of the early 20th-century movement depended on the widespread publicity provided by a group of journalists and writers who documented the "Death Roll of Industry." In an article on the dangers of various trades, one author charged that industrialists sent "to the hospital or the graveyard one worker every minute of the year."[7] One of the most graphic popular descriptions of the dangers of the meat packing industry was Upton Sinclair's *The Jungle* which detailed the close link between the exploitation of workers in the meat packing industry and the terrifying conditions of life for those living in the shadows of Chicago's meat packing district.[8]

Publicity for labor's plight was also provided by an extraordinary group of physicians, social activists, academics, and professionals such as Alice Hamilton, Paul Kellogg, and John R. Commons, who, as doctors, writers, lawyers, and social workers, were instrumental in popularizing this issue. They lectured, wrote articles, exposes, and books, sponsored meetings, and conducted independent investigations of conditions of Pennsylvania coal miners, Birmingham and Pittsburgh steel workers, New York City garment workers, Massachusetts textile workers, Minnesota iron miners, and numerous other industries.

Left-wing unions raised even more fundamental objections to the values and effects of business based civilization. "The average person is never tired of boasting about the wonderful achievements of modern civilization," noted a writer in *The Glass Worker* in 1908. "The huge factories dot the earth everywhere, polluting the landscape with their unsightly vomiting, but the question arises, are these mighty achievements worth the price that humanity is paying for them." *The Glass Worker* condemned modern capitalist industry and turned business rhetoric against itself: "The facts stand glaringly forth that social health and welfare are not being conserved. It is being forced into physical and moral bankruptcy because of the fearful price it has to pay for those achievements of which the average man is so boastful."[9]

One of the first and most important ways that muckrakers and other reformers sought to awaken the public to the horrible costs of industrialism was through popular discussion of the plight of women and children in mines, mills, and factories. Beginning in the late 19th century, magazines carried lurid stories of children awakening at dawn to toil at the looms, and women leaving their loved ones to work in the factory. By the early years of this century, there was hardly a journal that did not have articles that documented the special impact of industrialization for women and children. By 1900 over 1.7 million children worked for wages, many of them for 10 to 14 hours a day. Edwin Markham, a popular writer of the period, told of the little boys and girls who "sicken and faint" from "the heat and the odors ... in the fancy box and candy factories."[10]

The focus on women and children was a double-edged sword. It could be used to arouse the country to the dangers that all workers faced; it was also used to exclude female workers by asserting that it was wrong to subject the weaker sex to horrible working conditions.

To many at the turn of the century, worker safety and health was a primary source of conflict between workers and owners. The United States Commission on Industrial Relations found that dangerous and unhealthy working conditions were a crucial source of conflict and dissatisfaction in America. The commission also reported a widespread "fear ... of being driven to poverty by sickness, accident or involuntary loss of employment."[11]

Labor's anger at such conditions was frequently expressed in strikes at unhealthy and dangerous shops. One long and dramatic example of the discord created by dangerous health conditions was the nine-week general strike of cloak makers in New York City. The strike was called because of the "unsanitary condition in a large number of shops." The settlement, reached after the bitter and acrimonious picketing and public pressure, included the creation of a Joint Board of Sanitary Control. This body, composed of employers and employees, sought to establish sanitary standards for the industry. In one year the cloak makers union called 28 successful "sanitary" strikes in New York, and set the stage for the public outcry that followed the tragic deaths of 140 young women in New York's infamous Triangle Shirt Waist Fire in 1911.[12] (http://images.google.com/search?tbm=isch&hl=en&source=hp&biw=1899&bih=871&q=triangle+fire&gbv=2&aq=f&aqi=g10&aql=&oq=)

The horrible conditions that many workers faced every day led some socialists to call for revolution.[13] Such calls accelerated in the wake of the

Triangle Fire of March, 1911 when the country was galvanized by horrific pictures of young women jumping to their deaths from the loft building in which they worked and which had caught on fire. "When I read such records as this: 'Helper flooring factory-age 19 - clothing caught by setscrews in shafting; both arms and legs torn off; death ensued in five hours,' my spirit revolts," declared Crystal Eastman, the famous socialist spokeswoman in 1911. "And when the dead bodies of girls are found piled up against locked doors ... after a factory fire ... who wants to hear about a great relief fund? What we want is to start a revolution."[14]

The shock of the Triangle fire prompted many to indict industrial capitalists for their callousness and their greed. After a march and rally of 50,000 trade unionists, Rose Schneiderman, vice president of the Women's Trade Union League, argued, "I would be a traitor to these poor burned bodies if I came here to talk of good fellowship. The old Inquisition had its rack and thumb screws and its instruments of torture with iron teeth. We know what these things are today," she continued. "The iron teeth are the necessities, the thumb screws the high powered and swift machinery dose to which we must work, and the rack is here in the fire-trap structures that will destroy us the minute they will catch fire."[15]

The need to ameliorate the threat of class conflict and the nature of the problems that workers faced led to a broad conception of occupational safety and health. In the early years of the century labor joined with middle-class reformers to argue for a new definition of the intimate relationship between the health of workers and the health of the general community.

The most important example of this view of disease causation was contemporary discussion of tuberculosis, the devastating lung disease which ravaged working-class families, incapacitating children and grown-ups alike. In 1904, *Charities*, the journal of the Charity Organization Society, noted that tuberculosis, one of the worst scourges of the working classes, went hand-in hand with industrialism. It maintained that any effective program aimed at controlling the disease would have to acknowledge the relationship between home life, neighborhood, and workplace. Social workers and other professionals believed that tuberculosis struck those weakened by overwork, poor nutrition, or crowded living conditions. When these conditions were combined with a dusty work environment, a worker's health was almost sure to be impaired. An effective program, therefore, to control consumption required close attention to all aspects of a worker's life. For charity workers the issue of consumption illustrated the environmental, rather than the individual, roots of illness and dependence. "I would like to speak of the importance to the Charity Organization Society of health and safety conditions for labor," said Frederick Almy, secretary of Buffalo's chapter of the organization. "I think one-third or perhaps one-half of our work would disappear if labor conditions were all they might be. I mean if employers took as good care of their men as they do of their machinery."[16]

Social workers, forced by their experiences in the nation's growing slums, formed a *de facto* alliance with labor and turned to it for information and support. At the 25th Annual Convention of the American Federation of Labor in 1906, for instance, the delegates identified tuberculosis as one of its most pressing problems. In a dramatic chart showing the death rate from consumption in 53 occupations the A. F. of L. pointed out that stone cutters, cigar makers and plasterers, printers and servants all had death rates well above 4 per 1,000, while bankers, brokers, and officials had the lowest death rates, below 1 per 1,000. "All this means, really, the regulation of factory conditions, the regulation of housing, and the passage of child labor laws" was essential for battling the "Great White Plague."[17]

Union campaigns to make shop conditions more sanitary were linked to broader public health issues, most important, the battle against infectious disease. Cleaning up the workplace and keeping the workforce healthy were seen as benefits to both the worker and the public. In 1910 the greater New York local of the International Union of Bakers and Confectionary Workers conducted a successful strike to demand more sanitary working conditions. "Perhaps no phase of the trade union movement has ever affected the public so directly as the agitation for sanitary conditions in the bake shops," commented one leading periodical. In May of 1909, 3,000 Jewish bakers struck, and less than a year later 4,000 German workers followed suit. The union identified unsanitary workshops and the spread of infectious disease with nonunion bakeries. Their ability to link unsanitary working conditions to the health of the public gave their strike a tremendous appeal and power. [18]

Consumer groups also took up the issue of health conditions on the job and in the home. In part the appeal was based on fear, to make sure the middle class and wealthy would not be infected by goods tainted by sick workers. In the growing garment industry of New York, many dresses, shirts, and trousers were sewn on a piece-work basis in tenement slums, raising the specter that the same diseases infecting those in tenements would be transmitted to the men, women, and children of the middle class. Frances Perkins, who had served for two years as Secretary of the New York City Consumers

League also condemned the system of home work as "the most practical example which we have of the ability of industry to enslave its workers." But she also noted that this work also had a deleterious effect on public health: "One of the things which I noticed in regard to the system of this home work is that it is a menace to the health of the community and the health of the worker."[19]

The special social conditions surrounding work at the turn of the century led to the broad conception of the meaning of occupational safety and health. Occupational safety and health was part and parcel of a larger movement to reform American society. The movement to control workplace hazards was widespread, encompassing a variety of different groups. A wide variety of middle-class reformers and conservative labor representatives recognized that uncontrolled capitalism was killing and maiming so many workers that it was undermining the legitimacy of capitalism itself.

And this movement produced results: In little more than two decades, we saw the establishment of a meaningful federal Department of Labor, active women's and children's bureaus, the reinforcement and subsidization of state factory-inspection systems through state departments of labor, and the beginnings of a role in occupational safety and health within local health departments. We also saw the passage of the first significant child and women's labor legislation and a host of specific state acts regulating working conditions in tanneries, bakeries, foundries, and numerous other industries. Also, for the first time, there was a serious attempt to organize a more reliable method for collecting statistics on occupational injuries and deaths. Finally, it must be pointed out that in 1900 no state in the Union had a workers' compensation law. By 1915 every highly industrialized state had passed an act for some form of compensation. On the federal level, the reform movement was successful in passing a number of significant pieces of legislation. The railroad workers' compensation act in 1907 and a broader federal employees' compensation act were two of the landmark legislative efforts.

If the early 1900s were dominated by a concern over industrial accidents and acute poisonings from lead, phosphorus and other toxins in the mines, mills and foundries of industrializing America, the 1930s can be characterized as a period when the issue of long term disease began to emerge as a major issue among the workforce.

The Depression

The stock market crash of October, 1929 and the subsequent depression fundamentally altered many aspects of American life. With at least one quarter of the labor force unemployed and a much larger percentage of the population struggling to survive on reduced wages and the threat of layoffs, Americans had to confront a social and economic crisis of massive proportions. As you know, prior to 1933, there were no federal welfare programs, no social security payments, no unemployment benefits—no safety net to catch men and women, children and elderly, sick and disabled. What few social programs that did exist were run by private charity organizations, city welfare bureaus or state emergency relief agencies. Vast regions of the country did not even have minimal programs to support starving citizens in rural and urban communities. People were forced to develop their own networks for social support through families or friends. Workers and families organized self-help organizations, councils of the unemployed, and unions to find ways of controlling their own fate. They were forced to reformulate their assumptions about how to survive without work, social and familial support, or state or private mechanisms for guaranteeing basic necessities. Bread lines, riots, marches, rent strikes, sit-ins, and labor strife were the most obvious signs of the desperation of the times. But they also reflected the new range of options that working class Americans believed were legitimate for survival.[20]

Workers thrown out of work used any means necessary to survive and many workers in the dusty trades turned to the courts. Those who suspected that they were fired because of their impairments argued that industry bore the responsibility for their plight. They argued that their plight was not the result of individual failing or bad luck but was, rather, due to the inadequate protection offered them by their employers. The social crisis of the Depression created personal tragedies. But, as larger and larger numbers of workers in foundries and other silica industries turned to the courts for redress, their personal suffering became a national crisis. For the first time, the problem of chronic exposures and disease moved out of the domain of professionals and a few labor unions into the arenas of popular culture and public policy. Workers built a movement around the emerging union organizing efforts and the new CIO, demanding redress for the devastating effects that work had on their health.

Before the Depression would end, novels and movies, national magazine exposes and intense media attention would force the issue of industrially caused chronic disease onto the national agenda. The public now debated what had been the preserve of a small cadre of lawyers, doctors and public health professionals. Labor, management, industry and insurance representatives argued in terms accessible to laymen. During the Depression decade the very definition of disease was not the preserve of the elite but was part of a wider public dialogue. Many of the political and scientific battles took place around silicosis, a disease caused by the inhalation of dust produced in a wide variety of industries, in both urban and rural setting.

Workers in granite quarries in rural Vermont, in lead, gold, copper, zinc and silver mines in the west, foundries in numerous rural and urban settings and sandblasters, ubiquitous in a wide variety of construction or metal finishing plants all suffered from the disease. As late as 1929, silicosis had assumed a great deal of "importance in the minds of those concerned with public health" occasionally attracting the attention of a researcher or newspaper.[21] But, by and large, the issue remained below the radar until workers put out of work by the Depression began to push the issue themselves. By 1932, the head of New York State's Division of Industrial Hygiene, James Hackett, remarked on the strange dynamic which the public health community had become aware of the disease. Silicosis "would [have] continued to exist unnoticed in the community were it not for the fact that workers suffering from the disease, or the relatives of people who had died from the disease, have recently taken civil action against employers and have recovered considerable amounts of money therefore." The lawsuits brought "silicosis within the rage of practical politics."[22] By September, 1933, *Business Week* commented that an "epidemic of lawsuits" were "giving serious concern to the construction, quarry, and mining industries and to foundries and glass works...."[23]

Insurance companies were the first to understand the potential problems that the flood of lawsuits were creating because they were insuring foundries and other industries against liability suits through general comprehensive liability policies. One spokesperson for the industry argued that the problem was not that silicosis caused disability, but that unemployment caused workers to use the legal system as a welfare system and that unscrupulous lawyers were taking advantage of ignorant workers.[24]

The crisis for the insurance industry soon became a crisis for the various industries and the workforce as well. Insurance companies sought means by which to limit their risks through selectively insuring or cancelling industrial liability policies. High risk companies, such as foundries, metal mines, glass works, potteries and quarries were told that they had to examine all employees for signs of silicosis and to terminate those who showed any symptoms of disease. In the midst of the Depression when jobs were scarce, many of the employed were faced with unemployment if industry or insurance company physicians, utilizing x-rays, found suspicious signs of silicosis on the films. The effect of these new policies on the workforce was dramatic and immediate. Silicosis had become a social problem of immense proportions.

As social issues around silicosis entered the legal arena, professional disagreement, previously relegated to obscure technical journals, became a matter for contentious public debate. Because of the legal system's adversarial nature, the lawsuits highlighted the conflicting opinions of scientists, doctors and engineers about occupational lung diseases. Judges and juries, who in other circumstances would have preferred to defer to the "objective experts" in highly technical matters, found themselves in the position of having to decide which expert testimony to believe. Lawyers for workers and lawyers for insurance companies and industries each presented juries with their own groups of experts. Faced by conflicting medical testimony about the nature and causes of the plaintiff's lung condition, and faced with the worker's often obvious suffering, jurors in the early years of the Depression frequently brought judgments against insurance companies and industry alike. Because there were so many lawsuits especially in the industrial states and because so much hinged on the decisions of juries and judges, the public could see in a very concrete way that medical analysis and diagnoses were subject to conflicting interpretations and were the result of differing values and assumptions. Further, the fact that expert opinion could be bought by plaintiff and defendant alike demystified professional arguments. The very fact that foundries were such a ubiquitous part of America's industrial and agricultural base meant that friends and relatives of disabled foundry workers were educated about the workings of the professions.[25]

In the midst of the growing controversy over legal liability came the revelation that perhaps as many as 1,500 workers had been killed by exposure to silica dust while working on a tunnel project in Gauley Bridge, West Virginia. Newspapers and weeklies all over the country made silicosis a national scandal. In January, 1936, *Newsweek* wrote of "tunnelling through an atmosphere of deadly dust" and *Literary Digest* titled its article "Village of the Living Dead."[26] Now, silicosis was no longer the preserve of a small group of scientists, physicians, engineers and lawyers. It entered the popular lexicon. Even blues ballads of the era spoke of the meaning and horror of silicosis on the lives of hard rock miners, tunnellers and their families. Josh White, the well-known blues guitarist and folk singer, popularized "Silicosis Blues" in the 1936 where he spoke of the disease as a "robber and a thief" that "robbed me of my youth and health; all you brought poor me was misery." Another verse tells the story of Gauley Bridge: "I was diggin that tunnel for just six bits a day ... didn't know I was diggin my grave—silicosis was eatin my lungs away." Silicosis was seen as a broad social injustice: "Silicosis, you're a dirty robber and a thief ... robbed me of my right to live and all you brought poor me is grief." (http://www.youtube.com/watch?v=CjxCFYcCcNo)

Martin Cherniack, in his moving and authoritative book, *The Hawk's Nest Incident*, describes in detail the literary and epidemiologic evidence that led to public awareness of what he calls "America's worst industrial disaster." In his book he tells the story of the black and white workers who died of acute silicosis and other respiratory diseases while constructing this tunnel for the Union Carbide Company.[27]

In January and February, 1936, the Committee on Labor of the House of Representatives convened in order to consider a joint resolution "to authorize the Secretary of Labor to appoint a board of inquiry to ascertain the facts relating to health conditions of workers" employed by a subsidiary of "the Union Carbide and Carbon Company."[28]

In the course of the hearings witnesses testified that the workers had been placed at extraordinary risk while employed on the job. The 2000 workers were mostly southern rural Blacks drawn to the job and away from their families farther south by the promise of steady pay during the Depression. They had been ordered to drill through a mountain that was composed of nearly pure silica, even then known as a substance that destroyed lung tissue, incapacitating and killing its victims. Workers were sent into the tunnel despite widespread knowledge of the long-term dangers of silica dust and the recognition that only strict safety precautions such as wet-drilling, proper ventilation and masks could prevent massive exposure to silica dust. Workers complained that the company doctors told them they were suffering not from silicosis but from "tunnelitis," a fictitious condition meant to allay their fears.

The House Committee also heard testimony that company officials knew that they were systematically exposing workers to a disease that would eventually kill them. Company officials and engineers routinely wore masks when they entered the worksite. Furthermore, the company purposely bore through the site of the richest silica deposit so that silica rock and sand it could be shipped to another subsidiary of Union Carbide to be used in manufacturing.

Cherniack shows through a painstaking analysis of blueprints and engineering plans submitted to the state that the company altered the direction of their route through the tunnel in order to maximize the amount of silica that could be mined as a by-product.[29]

The impact of the incident itself and the revelations brought forth during the hearings was widespread within the labor community. *The American Federationist*, the official organ of the American Federation of Labor, editorialized that in addition to the hundreds known to have died, hundreds more could expect the worst.[30]

In part, this disaster was exposed because management did not expect the symptoms of silicosis to appear so quickly. Usually, the symptoms of silica poisoning, like the symptoms of asbestosis, brown and black lung disease, took years, if not decades, to appear. The long period between exposure and onset of symptoms would, therefore, obscure the company's role in their deaths. At Gauley Bridge, however, the extreme exposure to which workers were subjected caused the development of symptoms almost immediately. Workers were dying on the job, causing the company to hire a local undertaker to dispose of bodies in the fields nearby. The fact that the workers were primarily poor, Black migrants far away from their loved ones led management to believe that they could cover up the deaths. Families who inquired about the whereabouts of their husbands and sons were told that these men had "moved on." Despite testimony from workers, physicians, government officials and company doctors that showed the company's total disregard for the health of the workers, management still maintained a stony silence, maintaining that any disease was caused by workers' carelessness. Estimates of the number of affected workers varied greatly at the time. But Cherniack maintains that conservatively, more than 700 men died of silicosis and an untold number were diseased and disabled.[31]

As in the early progressive era movement, the insurance crisis and the popular attention to Gauley Bridge spurred the legislature of government to act. In 1936, the Department of Labor under Frances Perkins—who had begun her career as a factory inspector for New York State in the years following the Triangle fire—organized the first "National Silicosis Conference," bringing together representative of industry, labor and government to address the problem and Frances Perkins herself to descend into a mine to see first hand the conditions that created the disease.[32] The Labor Department produced one of its first films about the silciosis crisis, "Stop Silicosis," which documented both the social costs and causes of the disease to American workers.(http://www.youtube.com/watch?v=GtYErK9KjQ8) Sixty years later the disease was still a concern leading to federal conferences on how to stop this terrible scourge. It also remained a staple in verse and song. One song performed by Sweet Honey and the Rock, reminds us that the issue of occupational safety and health, and particularly silicosis, is not only of historical interest to workers and their families: "We bring more than a paycheck to our loved ones and families ... we bring Asbestosis, silicosis, brown lung, black lung disease and radiation hits the children before they've even been conceived.... I wanted more pay but what I've got today is more than I bargained for."(http://www.youtube.com/watch?v=UzlEGxiHpEU) This song certainly brings out the continuing importance of disease in the life of the American worker.

Notes

[1] Tony Mazzocchi, in "Proceedings," *Hazards of the Industrial Environment*, a conference sponsored by District 8 Council, Oil, Chemical and Atomic Workers International Union, Kenilworth, N.J., March 29, 1969, p.2.

[2] See as examples of this growing literature: Paul D. Blanc, *How Everyday Products Make People Sick : Toxins at Home and in the Workplace*, (Berkeley: University of California Press, 2007); Daniel Berman, *Death on the Job: Occuopational Safety and Health in the United States*, (New York: Monthly Review Press, 1978); Alan Derickson, *Black Lung: Anatomy of a Public Health Disaster,* (Ithaca: Cornell University Press, 1998); Alison Hepler, *Women in Labor: Mothers, Medicine and Occupational Health in the United States, 1890-1980*, (Columbus: Ohio State University Press, 2000); Christopher Sellers, *Hazards on the Job: From Industrial Disease to Environmental Health Science*, (Chapel Hill: University of North Carolina Press, 1997); Barbara Sicherman, *Alice Hamilton: A Life in Letters*, (Cambridge: Harvard University Press, 1984); Sarah Vogel, *Plastics, Politics and Production: the Political Economy of Bisphenol A,* (Berkeley: University of California Press, forthcoming, 2012).

[3] David Rosner and Gerald Markowitz, "The Early Movement for Occup0ationak Safety and Health, 1900-1917," in Judith Leavitt and Ronald Numbers, *Sickness and Health in America*, second edition, (Madison: University of Wisconsin Press, 1985),pp. 507-521.

[4] Arthur B. Reeve, "The Death Roll of Industry," *Charities and the Commons*, 17(1907), 791.
[5] Arthur B. Reeve, "The Death Roll of Industry," *Charities and the Commons*, 17(1907),791.
[6] Editorial, "Slaughter by Accident," *The Outlook*, 78(Oct. 8, 1904), 359.
[7] Arthur B. Reeve, "The Death Roll of Industry," *Charities and the Commons*, 17(1907),791.
[8] Upton Sinclair, *The Jungle*, (New York: Doubleday, Page & Co. 1906).
[9] "Is it Worth The Price?" *The Glassworker*, June, 2008, p.5.
[10] Quoted in Nora Gause, "The Slavery of Childhood," *The Woman's Label League Journal*, May, 1907, p.15.
[11] U.S. Commission on Industrial Relations, Preliminary Repiort," *The Survey*, 33(Dec. 12, 1914),288.
[12] "Joint Sanitary Standards in the Cloak, Suit, and Skirt Industry," *The Survey*, 26(Aug. 19, 1911),734.
[13] "Strikes for Good Health," *The Survey*, 27(Jan. 20, 1912),1592.
[14] Crystal Eastman, "The Three Essentials for Accident Prevention," *Annals of the American Academy of Political and social Sciences*, 38(June, 1911),98-99.
[15] "The Responsibility is on All Citizens," *The Survey*, 26(April 8, 1911),85.
[16] Frederick Almy, "Transcript of Proceedings, New York," *Second Report of the New York Factory Investigating Commission*, 1913, vol. iv, pp.1831-1832.
[17] "How to Prevent Consumption," *The International Woodworker*, 16 (May 1906), 137-139.
[18] "Investigations have Disclosed the Fact that Unhealthy and Poisonous Bread is Made in Non-Union Bake Shops," *The Woman's Label League Journal*, June, 1913, p.13.
[19] Frances Perkins, quoted in *Second Report of the New York Factory Investigating Commission*, Volume IV, pp.1576-1577.
[20] See, David Rosner and Gerald Markowitz, *Deadly Dust: Silicosis and the On-going Struggle to Protect Workers' Health*, Ann Arbor: University Press, 2006).
[21] "Silicosis Denounced as 'Murder' of Labor," *New York Times*, Mar. 7, 1929, p.4.
[22] James D. Hackett, "Silicosis," *New York Department of Labor Industrial Bulletin*, 11(Dec. 1932), 475.

[23] "Silicosis Menace," *Business Week*, Sept. 1933, pp.19-20.
[24] E.O. Jones to U.S. Department of Labor, Nov. 29, 1935, National Archives, Record Group 100, 7-2-1-5-1.
[25] See, David Rosner and Gerald Markowitz, *Deadly Dust: Silicosis and the On-going Struggle to Protect Workers' Health*, Ann Arbor: University Press, 2006), Chapter 3, pp.75-104.
[26] "Tunneling Through An Atmosphere of Deadly Dust," *Newsweek*, Jan. 25, 1936, p.33; "Village of the Living Dead," *Literary Digest*, Jan. 25, 1936, p.6.
[27] Martin Cherniack, *The Hawk's Nest Incident: Ameirca's Worst Industrial Disaster*, (New Haven: Yale University Press, 1986).
[28] U.S. Congress, House Subcommittee of the Committee on Labor, *An Investigation Relating to Health Conditions of Workers Employed in the Construction and Maintenance of Public Utilities*, 74th Cong., 2D Sess., Jan. 1936, Reprinted in Jim Comstock, ed. *West Virginia Heritage*, v. 7, Richwood, W.Va.: West Virginia Heritage Foundation, 1972, 1-3.
[29] Martin Cherniack, *The Hawk's Nest Incident: Ameirca's Worst Industrial Disaster*, (New Haven: Yale University Press, 1986).
[30] Editorial, *American Federationist*, 43(March 1936,), 245-246.
[31] Martin Cherniack, *The Hawk's Nest Incident: Ameirca's Worst Industrial Disaster*, (New Haven: Yale University Press, 1986).
[32] "National Silicosis Conference," *American Labor Legislation Review*, 26(1936),60.

Comment

Movements for Occupational and Environmental Health: History and Politics

Allison L. Hepler, Professor of History
University of Maine at Farmington, Farmington, Maine, USA

Two trends apparent in the first half of the 20th century likewise appeared in the second half. First, workplace health and safety in the past 60 years has continued to be shaped by the role of government. 1970 brought the federal Occupational Safety and Health Administration and a continued rise of expertise and bureaucratization of workplace safety and health. Second, broad-based social movements also appeared and prodded the nation forward in protecting workers' health, creating new practices in the workplace.

Specifically, since the 1960s, a number of groups emerged and, in some cases, created coalitions around issues of the workplace and the environment: broad-based environmental movement; unions, especially the United Automobile Workers and the Oil, Chemical and Atomic Workers Union; the women's movement, especially the women's health movement; and coalitions of workers, unions, health professionals with leftist sympathies, such as the Black Lung Association, which took charge when neither the United Mine Workers nor the company would move on black lung's effects on miners, and Committees on Occupational Safety and Health, or COSHs. In the few minutes that I have, I would like to speak about COSHs and the women's health movement.

COSHs, first formed in the mid-1970s in Chicago, were rooted in the New Left and civil rights politics of the Medical Committee on Human Rights in 1972. It quickly spread to many industrial cities, such as Philadelphia, New York, Buffalo, St. Louis, San Francisco and Los Angeles. People like Tony Mazzochi, president of the OCAW, actively sought coalitions between workers and environmentalists, telling environmentalists that they had to be involved with workers because they were the people on the front lines who suffered the worst. In fact, because environmentalists, labor activists, feminists, unions, socialists all had different agendas so it took people with good bridge-building skills and coalition-building skills. COSHs were also able to bridge those gaps between health professionals and unions, between unions and workers. In addition to Mazzochi, early leaders included Rick Engler, Dan Berman, and Joel Shufro.

The most successful and long-lasting COSHs were the ones that believed it was crucial to work within the labor movement and included unions, not just workers. Successful COSHs also created an effective working environment between middle-class health professionals with progressive politics but who saw unions as corrupt and working-class union activists who mistrusted industrial health people who they saw as either company employees or state bureaucrats who had little understanding of the shop floor.

COSHs had their work cut out for them because people who had come to be suspicious of each other had to come together. How did this work? Philaposh, for instance, persuaded rank and file dissidents within local unions that they had to work through the union. They also got health professionals (some of them medical students) in the same room with shop floor workers. Talking together broke down the mistrust and assumptions and the simple lack of knowledge about each other. Workers impressed by the health people's volunteerism and health professional volunteers learned about actual working conditions. The result was self-education—workers learned the technical terms they needed to talk back to their employers, no longer relying on outside employer experts. In many ways, COSHs developed an insider-outsider position in the fight for safer workplaces in the 1970s and 1980s. As the recipient of several grants from OSHA, they developed some legitimacy within the larger system of occupational safety and health. Yet they were also political activists, staging "sick outs" and picketing the homes of political leaders, happy to work outside the system of experts and collective bargaining.

The results were varied and two-pronged. As membership organizations, COSHs existed to provide advice and information to the workers and the local unions. With a significantly high level of volunteers, they shared information in newsletters, handbooks, hotlines, and conferences. Specific "fact sheets" explained hazards in plain terms. In demystifying the technical language of toxicology, COSHs provided new tools for workers to use against the bosses. COSHs also proved very effective at political action. Using the media to their advantage, Philaposh performed a "burial" of OSHA when President Ronald Reagan sought to drastically cut it in 1980. COSHs were also very good at using funds from OSHA, going to meetings sponsored by OSHA, and then criticizing them for inaction. Finally, in a move that has yet to receive significant scholarly attention from historians of workplace health and safety, "Right to Know" movements in cities and state across the country, in which the public asserted the right to know what hazardous materials were housed in its nearby factories, emerged in the 1980s. In many ways, this was the epitome of coalition-building. In Philadelphia, for instance, it connected fire fighters, neighborhood organizations, unions, and environmental organizations.

The women's health movement emerged about the same time, and it also affected workplace health and safety, albeit in a different way. This was also a product of self-education, of people coming together because they distrusted the "experts" in their lives, in this case mostly male physicians. For example, the Boston Women's Health Book Collective is well-known for its publication of the best-selling women's health handbook *Our Bodies Ourselves.* This group came together to gather and then share information on female health issues that had been ignored by the medical establishment. While some of what came out of this movement was personal health, the women's movement's call for more women in non-traditional jobs soon led to renewed concerns about the health of women in those jobs. On their own and in concert with organizations like COSHs, women activists held conferences, produced handbooks , and similar to COSHs, took government, unions, and employers to task—to their faces—about hazards. Leaders in this movement included Jeanne Mager Stellman, Wendy Chavkin, and Andrea Hricko.

One issue during this period was over "fetal protection policies," i.e., workplace policies that kept fertile women out of certain jobs that exposed them to reproductive hazards. What emerged as a result was a very interesting debate about women and workplace health that in many ways mirrored similar arguments from the early 20th century over sex-based protective labor legislation—should women be treated the same as men (equal protection and equal opportunity) or did women's reproductive capacity mean that women should be treated differently? From women's health activists in the 1970s and 1980s came the same sorts of arguments—and the same variety of perspectives—about working women's health that had come from Alice Hamilton, Florence Kelley, and Mary Anderson 100 years ago.

Some women's health activists argued that women's childbearing capacity was too often used to keep women out of high-paying jobs and that was neither fair nor right. With an emphasis on physical qualifications, activists argued that women should be free to choose whatever job they are qualified for. Others noted the biological rationale for protecting women: fetuses deserved special protection in the workplace (and only women had fetuses). Still others pointed out that the workplace should be cleaned up to protect mothers AND fathers. Health professionals disagreed over the best strategy and even over the best science. Indeed, it is clear that arguments over women's workplace health were never solely defined by medicine or science but by politics and by economics. Not surprisingly, the major argument from employers was economic: The Human Resources Director of Exxon said flatly that he'd rather face charges of sex discrimination than a deformed baby (injured pre-natally as a result of a workplace hazard). As a result, employers kept women out of certain jobs, and the US Supreme Court called them on it. In *UAW v. Johnson Controls* in 1991, the Court ruled it was unlawful sex discrimination to keep women out of those jobs. Left unsaid was any sort of protection for employers who might face that disabled baby. Left unsaid was also any mandate from the Court to make the workplace safe for all workers.

Another important contribution that the recent women's health movement has made to workplace health and safety has been new attention to office hazards—indoor air quality, chemicals from office equipment, ergonomics. And while men and women both share office space today, it is important to remember the gendered origins of this concern. One hundred years ago, reformist organizations like the National Consumers' League sought to improve the working conditions of women in department stores and telephone companies, and the proportion of women working in white-collar jobs has only increased in the years since. Also in this list should be efforts to clean up the hospital working environment, still a heavily female workplace.

Finally, as often happens, and as David Rosner and Gerald Markowitz have explained, reformers sometimes become part of the system, and this has been true of more recent movements as well; many activists in the areas of workplace health and women's health have moved into positions in public health, government, and academia, in some ways institutionalizing the changes they have sought.

Comment

Occupational Health Movements in France: History, Historiography and Politics

Laure Pitti
University Paris 8/CRESPPA-CSU
Paris, France

I AM DEEPLY honored to discuss David Rosner and Gerald Markowitz's keynote. First of all, I would like to thank the organizers, especially Paul Blanc, for inviting me to participate in this panel discussion to give, as he suggests, a "continental viewpoint," from a French perspective.

I would like to highlight two main points concerning the French history of occupational health and safety especially the history of social movements in this field.

1- How and when did French historians come to study occupational health issues?

French historical studies on occupational health issues are often considered separately from Anglo-Saxon historiography. This proves the importance of such international conferences to discuss similarities and differences between French and Anglo-Saxon histories and historiographies. In France, even if there is a long tradition of interest in occupational diseases especially among 19th century physicians—such as André Proust, Marcel Proust's father—the interest in this issue is relatively recent in French historiography. During the last decade, successively, this issue became important in three different fields: the history of work, workers and working conditions, the history of population and the history of migrations. The first studies on occupational health issues in France were carried out by social historians specialized in the field of work, workers and working conditions and not by the ones studying labor movements. Catherine Omnès who analyzed the careers of French female workers in Paris in the 20th century in her book *Ouvrières parisiennes. Marché du travail et trajectoires professionnelles au 20e siècle* (1997, EHESS Press) is one of these social historians. She then studied how physicians, ergonomists and other professionals contributed to the definition of work ability. This was the main subject of the book she published with Anne-Sophie Bruno in 2004: *Les mains inutiles. Inaptitude au travail et emploi en Europe* (Paris, Belin Publishers). In the same field, Nicolas Hatzfeld's research initially dealt with the history of assembly lines in the French Peugeot automobile factories and is now focusing on the history of musculoskeletal disorders that he tackled during the conference, but also in his article entitled "The Difficulty in the Recognition of Musculoskeletal Disorders between Transnational Medical Specialists, National Authorities and Social Players" published in the *Journal of Modern European History* in 2009.

Later on, occupational health issues started to interest French population historians. In his first book entitled *L'intelligence démographique: sciences et politiques des populations en France* published in 2003 by Odile Jacob, Paul-André Rosental studied the "Fondation Armand Carrel," as people generally called the French Foundation for the Study of Human Problems. This Foundation was created in 1941 under the Vichy regime with the aim of studying French population. He showed that this Foundation consisted of physicians and hygienists more than demographers; and thus highlighted the links between public health policy and population policy at that time. This partly explains how Paul-André Rosental came to study the history of silicosis as an occupational disease in France and at a transnational level ("Health and Safety at Work. A Transnational History," *Journal of Modern European History*, published by Rosental in 2009). He then conducted a more thorough research on the French history of occupational health in general and published *La santé au travail, 1880-2006* (2006, La Découverte) together with Stéphane Buzzi and Jean-Claude Devinck, two other historians.

Furthermore, the historiography of silicosis became important at an international level thanks to Bernard Thomann's research on the history of silicosis in Japan. Japan is therefore a prolific field for French researchers who work on the history of occupational and environmental health. In his book *Maladies industrielles et renouveau syndical au Japon* (2006, EHESS Press), the French sociologist Paul Jobin focused on the "Minamata disease" and disaster in Japan. It is important to note that this kind of approach regarding occupational and environmental diseases are still rare in French historiography with the exception of a few recent studies such as the one carried out by Thomas Le Roux on craft and industrial pollution at the end of the 18th Century and in the beginning of the 19th Century (that will be published by Armand Colin in 2011).

At a later time, occupational health issues became an important subject of study in the field of the history of migrations. This is not very surprising as migrant workers were highly exposed to and thus mainly concerned by occupational diseases. French social historians started to research on European or colonial migrations. Judith Rainhorn studied Italian migrations, Anne-Sophie Bruno focused on Tunisian migrations while I carried out research on Algerian migrations. Moreover, in the past few years we have been studying lead poisoning in the workplace with Judith Rainborn focusing on the early 20th Century and myself on the second half of the 20th Century. Anne-Sophie Bruno is researching on work ability and inability. Even though the French historiography of occupational health is relatively recent, it is becoming increasingly prolific.

2- French and American occupational health history: comparative approach to prevention in the workplace

In the area of occupational health policies, we will highlight the issues of compensation and prevention in the workplace and the social players who contributed to their emergence to analyze the differences between France and the US. In France, the compensation system was early established by the 1898 Act related to occupational hazards and the 1919 Act setting out the legal framework for occupational disease recognition. However, from that time, professionals in the field such as occupational physicians or ergonomists focused on work ability—and not on prevention in the workplace. As a matter of course, occupational health doctors have been working legally in French factories since 1946. According to the 1946 Act, they were employed to legally protect the health of workers from any damage caused by their work. However, if they had no time to dedicate to observing working conditions until 1969, how could they efficiently protect workers' health? This is extremely different from what David Rosner and Gerald Markowitz describe when giving the example of Dr. Alice Hamilton's inquiries in the beginning of the 20th century and their contribution to the publicity for labor's plight. Nonetheless, later on, the 1960s and 70s were a turning point for both the French (and European) and the American history of occupational health. At that time, the compensatory model of occupational hazards and accidents was deeply challenged in several European countries.

On the one hand, in a "bottom-up" historical perspective, this compensatory model was challenged by several strikes in France but also in Italy in the wake of the 1968 social movement (1969 in Italy).The most important thing to observe in these strikes is that workers contested the compensation system with a main slogan: "*Our health is not for sale*" used both in Italy and in France. It is also important to note that at that time such protests against lead poisoning and asbestos were organized by the workers themselves and not by trade unions. As Ronnie Johnston pointed out in this conference, these kind of protests show the importance of lay knowledge on occupational health at that time.

Social actors played an increasingly important role: scholars like the toxicologist Henri Pézerat in France or the psycho-sociologist Ivar Oddone in Italy were particularly involved in such protests. Figuratively speaking, they were a bridge between workers and companies or between workers and administration putting this lay knowledge into value.

On the other hand, from a transnational perspective, it is also very interesting to analyze the effects that the establishment of the Council of the European Communities might have had on this history of occupational disease prevention. This can be compared to the crucial role played by American federal administrations or agencies at that time, such as the Occupational Safety and Health Administration studied by Rosner and Markowtiz or the Environmental Public Agency. In fact, in 1972, both the CEC and the American EPA organized an international conference on lead poisoning. In Europe, this conference was a first step towards the enactment of the Council Directive of the 3rd December 1982 on a limit value for lead in the air—*for the very first time*. The French administration was obliged to apply this directive and tried to resist. Yet, the limit value was finally adopted in 1988. As David Rosner and Gerald Markowtiz point out with regards to federal legislation, the French history of prevention in the workplace has to be taken into consideration not only on the national but also on the European and the transnational level.

Comment

Building on the Past

Joseph Melling
Center for Medical History
University of Exeter, Exeter, UK

I BEGIN BY saying that the scholarship of David Rosner and Gerry Markowitz has been one of the reasons why I became interested in the history of occupational health and of dust at work and he has shown me once again why I have long been so impressed with their intellectual passion and their breadth of historical understanding.

David echoes Mazzocchi's comment that we have a moral responsibility as historians to retrieve from history the struggles of workers from the past and place it alongside an official record that often denied the validity and significance of these movements.

This is fundamentally a valid point but my question for David and this conference is "where do we go from here?" It is not that the critical perspective has triumphed over conservative views or that radical resistance to business hegemony and official proceduralism is no longer needed. It is. But how do we recognised the relationship of knowledge and understanding in different social and political worlds: how do we explain differences within the scientific community and between labour activists, environmentalists, radical ecologists, strategic conservatives, concerned consumers and all the people that Chris Sellers mentioned in his overview. More importantly, what moral choices can we and should we make about other countries—such as China or Mexico—which provide the goods that we use and whose workers often experience the kind of poisoning that we have heard about in smelting plants and even in restaurants and bars not to mention other forms of human exploitation. So my question is about how we write a history of difficult choices and I have three specific comments that David may wish to respond to.

The first one echoes Christine Rosen's comment on Chris Sellers yesterday and it could be simply phrased as many of my medical colleagues have done without fear of being denounced as presentists—namely, what would have made for a good business culture at the time? What solutions were made and should have been made more widely? Some employers were known as good employers and even Gabriel Kolko many years ago suggested that many business leaders were pro-reform for a mixture of instrumental and strategic reasons. Is there a model of good business practice that we should see as a trend setter?

Secondly and related to this point, was state regulation the only effective option and was it the preferred option of organised labour on every issue? If states regulate then should labour organisations and environmental groups rely on governments to monitor toxins and pollution? What we have heard quite a lot about at the conference is the difficulty of building a secure coalition for reform and good practice. In particular we have potential constituencies of industry, local community, and consumers, leaving aside the question of the wider environment. David shows how there could be and sometimes were important alliances between the different constituencies and he shows us how activists could make common cause with the progressives but there are also conflicts—as we know from studies of oil industry and chemical plants in different parts of the world, groups in civil society and in political worlds often have influence they use for specific interests so how would a coalition sustain itself—as we heard in discussions of OHSA and NIOSH, there are often conflicts about ends and means.

Thirdly, people at this conference have shown how the hazards move around and are changing over time and that many of the heroic struggles we see in David's case study of dust are not as easy where modern worklife problems are associated. I am involved in a new project on the history of workplace stress in the UK and other countries and what we see there is that the terms of the problem have remained contested even though it is now widely claimed that stress is the single greatest cause of the loss of days of work and efficiency in industry throughout the developed and possibly developing worlds. So the question becomes how do we construct the kind of narrative that David has presented here for other less easily-defined problems where material concerns exist but material evidence is often difficult to detect.

The paper stresses the importance of a clear economic and political context for understanding occupational hazard. The growing concern over safety and health issues in the first decade of the 20th century arose in the wake of the revolutionary social and economic changes that America had just undergone. In little more than three decades Americans had witnessed the virtual explosion of urban and manufacturing centers. This was shocking to Americans reared in rural settings. Before the Civil War, most Americans lived on farms or in small towns; the few factories that existed were scattered in mill towns and villages in the Northeast. With the growth of the transcontinental railroads, however, the development of national markets, increased exploitation of natural resources such as coal and iron, and the massive immigration of labor from rural Europe to the cities of the East and Midwest, conditions of work changed dramatically. America moved from being a fourth-rate industrial power to the leading industrial producer in the world. But work for the vast majority of laborers deteriorated. Speed-ups, monotonous tasks, exposure to chemical toxins, metallic and organic dusts, and unprotected machinery made the American workplace among the most dangerous in the world. In mining, for instance, England, Germany, and France experienced death rates of fewer than 1.5 per 1,000 workers during the first years of this century. In the United States more than 3 miners in every 1,000 could expect to die while working in a mine during any given year. The enormous wealth produced by the new industrial plants was achieved at an inordinate social cost. All this provides a vivid context for the kind of arguments outlined in studies of silicosis dangers.

My overall impression is that we can now build on the work of David and Gerry to extend the debate towards the question of multiple agency in the reconstruction of health and safety agendas around issues of dust and other toxic environments. We know that in some instances workers sought to protect their own privileges and interests at the expense not only of the enterprise which often exposed them to dangerous circumstances, but also in over-riding the concerns of other, often less secure, workers. The decision to struggle always involve moral choices within cultural codes that may advantage some people over others and may be deeply contested for labor as well as capital.

This leads to the recognition that scientists and technicians may be considered intellectual laborers who were themselves divided by responsibility and by orientation and ethical perspective in responding to the evidence of hazards faced by other workers. The most senior scientists were usually protected by professional associations and networks that frequently extended to government, though whether or not there was a drive to "objectivity" at the expense of empathy in the mid-20th century must remain a matter of discussion. David and Gerry usefully note a growing concern with technical measurement rather than human subjective responses in the United States during the 1940s-50s (with honourable exceptions), though again these moves were colored by political and social pressures of the period and the loyalties of the individuals concerned. It can be argued that in the Cold War years there was a growing conservatism among many leading scientists as well as union leaders, but in the 1960s-70s there was a resurgence of interest in occupational risks led by notable network-builders as Selikoff in the United States. In the U.K. the scientific community possessed a stronger core of left-inclining occupational health experts from the 1930s onwards.

The thread that binds these themes together in the growing internationalisation of knowledge about occupational illness from the 1930s conferences on silicosis to the 1960s-70s congregations dealing with asbestos dangers. These events reflected the changing political concerns of states facing with populations capable of challenging governments as well as employers in the courts and a mass media that found the environmental threats posed by production to be highly newsworthy.

Keynote

Occupational Disease and Labor Health and Safety Under the Nazis

Robert N. Proctor
Stanford University, Palo Alto, CA, USA

(Please note - see medicalhumanities.ucsf.edu/book-series for link to accompanying PowerPoint slides of images referred to in the text.)

We tend to think about efforts to improve occupational health and safety as a good thing, which is one reason I think people are surprised to learn about Nazi efforts to safeguard worker health and safety. Nazi doctors spent a great deal of time trying to identify and reduce exposures to asbestos and tobacco smoke and radioactive isotopes; and indeed in several of these areas for a time at least, Germany led the world.[1] The Nazis wanted a strong and productive workforce; they also took steps to limit exposure of women and children to certain toxics, part of a broader effort to safeguard "the German national body" and "the German germ plasm." Hitler himself was regarded as "the doctor of the German people," and Nazism the solution to all its ills (See Figure 1 of PowerPoint). Hitler promised to put an end to Germany's joblessness and political squabbling; his party also had the advantage of not scaring off big business: when asked whether he would nationalize industry, Hitler gave a very interesting answer: "why nationalize industry when you can nationalize the people?"

Labor held a special aura for the Nazis, though in a somewhat different way from, say, the Stakhanovites of Soviet Russia or radicals in the Americas: work was not so much a right as a "duty," comparable to military service or, for women, the bearing and rearing of children. In May of 1933 an IG Farben food chemist and long-standing Nazi by the name of Robert Ley engineered a coup d'etat against the unions, following which all workers were required to join the newly-formed German Labor Front, a factory policing agency with unprecedented powers over life in the workplace. The German Labor Front was supposed to make Germans "the healthiest, high-performance people in the world." Performance medicine and selection medicine were supposed to raise productivity by improving the work environment and weeding out the weak or recalcitrant. Hand labor and brain labor were also supposed to be united (Figure 2). Performance-enhancing drugs were part of this, which is why so many Germans in the Nazi era became addicted to amphetamines.

War mobilization was crucial here. The four-year plan announced in 1936 put all of German production on a military footing, increasing both the pace of work and the number of hours put in. Many industries ended up demanding sixty hour work weeks, which dramatically increased the number of accidents and injuries, dutifully recorded in the many professional journals devoted to labor medicine (see Table, end of chapter). Nazi officials put an unprecedented number of physicians on factory floors—with the goal of supervising health and safety, but also to certify who was sick and to identify shirkers. The number of "factory physicians" grew from only 467 in 1939 to an astonishing 8,000 in 1944, having as their job assignment the maintenance of labor discipline and whatever else was needed to ensure optimal employee performance.

Here I want to look at how Nazi authorities wrestled with several of the most notorious occupational carcinogens from this era: cancers caused by X-rays, exposure to radium and uranium, and exposures to arsenic, asbestos, and aniline dyes. I should also note that I first became interested in this topic working on my book, *Racial Hygiene*, and explored it further in my *Nazi War on Cancer*, where I was especially interested in exploring the milieu that gave rise to the great Wilhelm Hueper.

The take-home message is that Nazi health protections have to be understood in the context of racism, militarism, anti-feminism, and a productivist "performance ethic" that subordinated whatever protections were put into place to the exigencies of total war. I also think we have to realize, though, that the development of a state of perpetual emergency compromised many of the health protections advanced by the regime, and that the defeat of the Reich caused much of this all to be forgotten.

Roentgen-Rays

X-radiation was discovered in 1895, and by the turn of the century the "wonder rays" had already found uses in hundreds of clinical settings. X-rays were used to combat hysteria and infertility, and even to precipitate hair loss so that other diseases (like ringworm) could be treated. Worries about a cancer hazard emerged in the first decade of the twentieth century, with skin cancers of the hand the first to be noticed—especially among X-ray technicians, who often tested the rays with their hands. German physicians published evidence of X-ray-induced breast cancer in 1919, uterine and cervical cancer in 1923, and bone cancer in 1930. By the end of the 1920s there was a sizeable literature on radiation carcinogenesis, including a large body of work based on animal experiments.

Reports that X-rays could cause genetic damage began to be taken seriously in the 1920s, especially by eugenicists. Sterility amongst X-ray workers started to be noticed, along with deformities in newborn babies. Racial hygienists like Fritz Lenz and Eugen Fischer were among the loudest in sounding the alarm, leading the Bavarian Society for Pediatrics to adopt a resolution—in 1927—recommending that pregnant women receiving X-ray treatments should abort their fetuses. Fischer in 1930 warned that exposed women should be permanently barred from bearing children, and his colleagues at the Institute for Anthropology in Berlin proposed the construction of an "archive of irradiated girls and women" to identify and counsel such women against having children.

Eugenicists' worries in this realm have to be understood in light of the fact that many physicians displayed a rather cavalier attitude towards radiation safety. Negligence was propelled by the fact that radiologists and radiotherapists were far more interested in promoting X-rays than in warning against harms; indeed, when it came to the question of whether to warn the public about possible long-term genetic damage, professional radiological societies were very clearly opposed. In 1931, when the German Genetics Society and Society for Racial Hygiene warned that X-rays could cause genetic damage, the Bavarian Society for Roentgenology produced a sharply-worded rebuttal, claiming that the evidence of hazards was based only on "experimental studies of insects and plants." Radiotherapists characterized it as "extremely dangerous" to raise the specter of radiation hazards, given that one might impede the advance of X-ray therapeutics and diagnostics.

All of this was interestingly politicized, and in ways that to today's ears might sound upside down. Radiologists had allies in defense of radiation amongst the leaders of the Association of Socialist Physicians, Germany's most prominent left-wing medical association; socialist physicians were among the earliest critics of Nazi racial hygiene; strange today, however, is their ridicule of the specter of long-term health damage from X-rays as yet another instance of racial scare-mongering. Julian Marcuse, writing in 1932 in the association's journal, derided the Nazi distrust of X-rays as "racial fanaticism," one of the first uses of this expression in the Nazi context.

The fact that Nazi racial hygienists came out on the "right" side of the X-ray/genetic damage issue may be surprising, but we should also realize there were conflicting agendas even within the Nazi Party about how bad it was to be exposed to radiation. One of the biggest fears at this time was of tuberculosis—the second leading cause of death in Germany until the mid-1920s. Fear of TB was one reason Nazi officials demanded mass X-ray screenings—of everyone in a factory or an entire student body—to identify potential carriers. On August 5, 1933, the *Deutsches Ärzteblatt*—basically the *JAMA* of Germany--reported on a new rule at the University of Munich that all students be X-rayed. Sixty students were found to be infected (among 1,000 screened) and barred from university classrooms. Similar exams were required at other German universities and at the Nuremberg party congress of 1938, assembled dignitaries all lined up to have themselves X-rayed. (Figure 3) One SS roentgenologist personally administered 10,500 X-rays to SS men over a six-day period, and mobile X-ray units were deployed at German factories to screen workers for silicosis.

The net effect: despite warnings about dangerous levels of exposure by racial hygienists, the number of people X-rayed increased dramatically under the Nazis. The SS established special "X-ray battalions" with special X-ray bulbs and films to speed up screening, which led to vans that had the capacity to X-ray up to 600 people per hour—one every six seconds. Germany becomes "the most X-rayed nation in the world," and not just for TB, cancer, and silicosis, but also for heart disease, stomach ailments, asbestosis, circulatory problems, and other diseases. The process took on a quasi-military character during the war, when medical authorities sought to identify and isolate infirm workers. Soldiers and civilians were X-rayed on the eastern front, and mass screenings were used to identify tubercular Poles, one of the first victims of the mass murders after Hitler's invasion in September of 1939.

A particularly brutal use of X-rays emerged in Auschwitz, where experiments were performed to determine whether X-rays might be used to prevent the breeding of Jews: SS Oberführer Viktor Brack proposed the sterilization of Europe's Jewry in a letter to Himmler of June 23, 1942:

> Among 10 millions of Jews in Europe there are, I guess, at least 2-3 millions of men and women who are fit enough to work. Considering the extraordinary difficulties the labor problem presents us with, I hold the view that those 2-3 millions should be specially selected and preserved. This can, however, only be done if at the same time they are rendered incapable to propagate. About a year ago I reported to you that agents of mine had completed the experiments necessary for this purpose. I would like to recall these facts once more. Sterilization, as normally performed on persons with hereditary diseases, is here out of the question, because it takes too long and is too expensive. Castration by X-ray however is not only relatively cheap, but can also be performed on many thousands in the shortest time.[2]

Brack had earlier proposed that X-ray sterilization (castration) could be done surreptitiously:

> One practical way of proceeding would be, for instance, to let the persons to be treated approach a counter, where they could be asked to answer some questions or to fill in forms, which would take them 2 or 3 minutes. The official sitting behind the counter could operate the installation in such a way as to turn a switch which would activate the two valves simultaneously (since the radiation has to operate from both sides). With a two-valve installation about 150-200 persons could then be sterilized per day, and therefore, with 20 such installations as many as 3,000-4,000 persons per day.[3]

Brack's grandiose scheme was never implemented; a series of experiments at Auschwitz by the gynecologist Horst Schumann determined that the people sterilized by this method were burned so severely they were no longer capable of work. Nearly all of the subjects of these experiments--at least a hundred people--were later killed.

For healthy Germans, however, practical steps were taken to limit X-ray exposures, with the "X-Ray Ordinance" issued by the Labor Ministry on February 7, 1941 establishing an occupational tolerance of .25 roentgen per day, with a tolerance dose ten times stricter (.025 roentgen per day) "when there is a possibility of genetic damage." German regulations may have been more strictly followed than elsewhere, judging from the massive outpouring of compliance literature produced in the wake of the law, detailing optimal levels of shielding, control of beam coherence, and so forth.

Radium and Uranium

"Radioactivity" was discovered at the end of the nineteenth century and soon thereafter launched as a medical fad, with radium salts incorporated into spa waters, radium bandages, inserts in shoes, radium bath tablets, radium creams, and my favorite: radium cigarettes (see Figure 4). Inhalation therapies were designed to mimic the vapors of radioactive baths, and radioactive tonics were sold along with mesothorium-impregnated milk sugar and even radium-infused chocolate.

One reason medical professionals may have been slow to appreciate the hazards of radioactivity is that German spas were heavily invested in promoting the curative virtues of radiation. Therapeutic baths were a vital part of upper middle-class conceptions of healing--and the discovery of "radioactive emanation" in the water of many of these spas led to a belief that radon must be the therapeutic agent. Millions of Germans traveled to radioactive spas in the first half of the twentieth century, hoping to be revitalized by the experience. (Some of these are still open today, with just as much radon to inhale.) Spa health physicists were organized and powerful, and tended to argue that radioactivity in this form was more likely to heal the body than to harm it. Elaborate theories were put forward to explain how radon enlivened the body: a 1938 review, for example, claimed that the radioactive gas promoted "oxidation" and "stimulate[d] cells and tissues without injuring them very much." Radon therapy was described as "a special form of shock therapy," awakening and augmenting the body's own natural healing powers.[4]

We're all familiar with the poisonings suffered by the American radium dial painters; luminous dial painting was important in Germany, too, especially when blackouts were imposed with allied bombing. Fewer women seem to have been affected, however, because German women did not "point" their brushes in their mouths.

The largest occupational cancer hazard from radioactivity, however, was that faced by *miners*, especially the uranium-cobalt-silver miners in and around the town of Schneeberg and Joachimsthal (Jachymov), near the Czechoslovakian border. The "Ore Mountains" south of Dresden had long been mined for rare metals: that in fact is where we get the name "dollar," which is shortened from Joachimsthaler, a coin renowned for its high grade of silver (Figure 5). Schneeberg's were the first clinically-diagnosed occupational lung cancers, documented already in the 1870s, though no one yet suspected radiation. Epidemiologists in 1926 showed that nearly three quarters of the miners in the region were dying from lung cancer—which prompted the Weimar government to classify the *Schneeberger Krankheit* as a compensable occupational illness. Experts blamed TB germs or arsenic or silica dust or molds from rotting mine shaft supports, and the disease was not nailed down as radiogenic until the 1930s.

Interest in the *Schneeberger Krankheit* was renewed in 1933, when the mines were reopened in anticipation of a Nazi-inspired economic recovery. Boris Rajewsky, Director of Frankfurt's Institute for the Physical Foundations of Medicine and a health and safety officer in Germany's atom bomb project, showed that radiation in the air of the mines was often on the order of 10,000 pCi/l—an extraordinary level. The Labor Ministry concluded that long term work in air containing even far lower levels of radon could be dangerous: experiments were done to determine how much radioactivity was present in the urine and exhaled air of miners—also to determine how the radioactivity of the air varied with changing weather conditions.[5]

Experiments were also performed which produced lung cancers in animals raised in the mines. Julius Löwy in 1929 had shown that the disease faced by Joachimsthal miners was the same as the *Schneeberger Krankheit*, but it was not until 1938 Arthur Brandt, an industrial physician working for the government in Dresden, was able to reproduce the cancer hazard under laboratory conditions. His results, published in 1938, showed that twenty-five percent of the mice raised for one year in the shafts evidenced tumors upon dissection. This was the first conclusive animal experimental evidence of a lung cancer hazard from breathing air in the mines, and proof for many that inhaled radioactivity was the most likely cause of the *Schneeberger Krankheit*.

It is first in the Nazi era that we find this consensus that radioactivity was causing the lung cancers of Germany's uranium (and silver) miners. The chief physician of the German Labor Front, Hermann Hebestreit, stated unequivocally in a 1939 review that "the lung cancer of the Joachimsthal uranium miners is traceable to exposure to radioactive materials." Germans were the first to recognize this fact; American health officials as late as the 1950s, by contrast, were still questioning the link. German uranium miners were in fact obtaining compensation for occupational lung cancers by the end of the 1920s; Americans had to wait until the passage of the Radiation Exposure Compensation Act in 1991.[6]

Nazi ideology, of course, placed a higher value on certain people's health than others, and this can be seen in correspondence concerning whom to employ in the mines. On November 19, 1938, SS Oberführer and Regierungspräsident Hans Krebs wrote to Himmler, asking him to install concentration camp prisoners in Joachimsthal to free "our poor Sudeten German miners" from work that was killing them in their 40s. Himmler agreed on the condition that the prisoners be released after 2-3 years if they showed good conduct, though it is not yet clear whether such proposals were ever implemented.[7]

One thing we do know is that tens of thousands of political prisoners—many of them former Nazis—worked in the Joachimsthal mines after the war, producing 90,000 tons of uranium for the Soviet atomic arsenal and many thousands of deaths from lung cancer. The Schneeberg mines generated an estimated 200,000 tons for the Soviet nuclear effort. These were enormous undertakings: by 1949 the uranium mining operation in East Germany alone (code-named *Wismut*—literally "bismuth") employed 80,000 men and women, many of whom had started work as forced laborers. More than half a million people eventually toiled for *Wismut* at one time or another, until the unification of Germany in 1989 closed most of the shafts.

Schneeberg is now the target of Europe's largest environmental cleanup, one of many environmental nightmares inherited from the Cold War. In the early 1990s the director of Germany's Federal Office of Radiation Protection estimated an eventual death toll among miners in the region of 10,000 to 15,000 from radiation-induced lung cancer, and perhaps twice this many from silicosis.

Another interesting aspect of this story is that the Americans who occupied the area in 1945 were seemingly unaware of its military significance. American officials seem to have overlooked the uranium in the region, perhaps because the abortive German atomic bomb project had neglected domestic sources in favor of Belgian Congo deposits.

The oversight is curious, given that fear of German control of the Joachimsthal mines had originally stimulated Albert Einstein to draft his famous letter to President Roosevelt about the possibility of a Nazi bomb. Compounding the oddity is the fact that J. Robert Oppenheimer, the man chosen to coordinate the Manhattan Project had actually written his senior thesis at the Ethical Culture School in New York on the mines at Joachimthal. Joachimsthal had monopolized the world's supply of radium prior to the First World War—making it strange indeed that U.S. authorities missed its atomic potential. Soviet officials were more astute: geologists were sent to Schneeberg to prospect for uranium in June of 1945, and shortly thereafter acquired control over the region in exchange for giving up West Berlin.

American military officials must have eventually regretted the oversight: in 1953, AEC Chairman Gordon Dean wrote that the Joachimsthal mines alone "could support a sizeable sizeable atomic energy program."[8]

Asbestos

There are many other occupational hazards explored in this era. The Nazi Party Chancellery banned the use of arsenic pesticides in February of 1942, for example, allowing vintners to use up their stocks by June 30, 1942. Vintners had earlier been barred from applying compounds containing lead. German industrial hygienists recognized that while exposure to any dust was harmful, the worst in terms of the numbers of people affected was probably quartz or silica dust. Silicosis—the German is *Quarzstaublunge*, literally "quartz dust lung"—was regarded as the king of occupational lung disease, killing more, it was said (and perhaps rightly so) than all other dusts combined. Hundreds of scientific articles on the topic can be found in the German medical literature of the 1930s, describing everything from the maximally hazardous particle size to a possible cancer link. Gauley Bridge played a big role for Germans, and the hope was that avoid such catastrophes. Safeguards put into place, and from 1929 through the end of the 1930s, more than sixty million Reichsmarks had been paid to silicotic workers or their relatives in accordance with Germany's occupational health and safety laws.

Steps were taken early in the Nazi era to combat dust diseases in German industry. On April 4, 1934, a Dust Control Office was established by the quarryman's union to coordinate the struggle; the office explored new ways of constructing hoods and vacuum devices, and new kinds of filters and ventilators. In Thuringia, the office worked with the slate roofing industry to lower the dust involved in splitting slate and the dust inhaled by stonemasons handling sand and cement. Synthetics abrasives were developed, and scuba-like breathing gear was introduced for sandblasting. A journal devoted to research in the area of dust control technology was established in 1936 (*Staub: Reinhaltung der Luft*); the journal continued publishing until 1943, and was continued after the war by the Dust Research Institute of Dusseldorf.

One of the most remarkable aspects of dust research in this era was the recognition of a cancer hazard from asbestos. The first modern medical description of asbestosis dates from England in the nineteenth century, though German asbestosis fatalities were not identified until 1914, by which time English and American interest in the topic was already well underway. Germans tended to manufacture finished asbestos products, which is how workers there first began to contract the disease. Asbestos in these early years was commonly referred to as *Bergflachs*—literally "mountain flax"—and asbestosis soon became known as *Bergflachslunge* or "mountain flax lung," a rather rustic euphemism for such a devastating scourge.

The possibility of a cancer hazard was not suspected until the 1930s, by which time tens of thousands of workers—especially in the shipbuilding industry—were routinely handling the fiber. Naval officials were intrigued by its insulating and fire-resistant properties: asbestos was used to insulate steam pipes and to seal and fireproof steam-engine boilers. Asbestos was used for brake shoes and clutch facings; it was also used to strengthen cement, to fireproof paints and textiles, and to render roofing and floor tiles fire-resistant.

Recognition of a cancer hazard came in 1938, when three German papers and an Austrian review provided strong evidence of a link.[9] An occasional association of asbestos and lung cancer had earlier been reported in both England and America, but the German reports were the most comprehensive. Franz Koelsch in his contribution noted that the twelve lung cancers thus far tied to asbestosis did not absolutely prove the link, but others were not so reticent. Ludwig Teleky in Vienna reasoned that it was "extremely likely" that asbestosis was a predisposing factor for lung cancer. The Hanover pathologist Martin Nordmann made the strongest case of the lot, identifying lung cancer as an established hazard of asbestos workers, afflicting roughly twelve percent of those who suffer from asbestosis. Nordmann concluded that "a new occupational cancer" had arrived in Germany.

By this time, German labor authorities had already taken steps to reduce the risk posed to workers handling the fiber. Asbestos was a major target of an "anti-dust campaign" launched in 1936. New kinds of ventilators were introduced, and the dustiest jobs were moved to hoods where dust could be drawn away from the workplace.

Recognition of a lung cancer hazard spurred occupational authorities to strengthen dust exposure standards. On August 1, 1940, the Asbestosis Committee founded by the Labor Ministry in collaboration with the German Society for Labor Protection issued formal guidelines specifying acceptable levels of dust and techniques to be used in its reduction. The guidelines barred anyone under eighteen from working with the fiber and reaffirmed the cancer danger.[10] Research also continued into the mechanisms of carcinogenesis, including use of Siemens newly-invented *Übermikroskop* (Figure 6). A 1942 article by a Hanover colleague of Nordmann reported a lung cancer in a worker who had worked only four years with the fiber; and 1943 Hans-Wilfried Wedler of Berlin published a paper showing that asbestos workers were prone to suffer from mesothelioma—also incorporated into medical textbooks.[11]

Animal experiments were also used to document the asbestos-lung cancer link. In 1941, Nordmann and his Hanover colleague, Adolf Sorge (a Nazi party member and SS officer), exposed a group of mice to asbestos dust over a period of several weeks and found that twenty percent of the survivors had developed tumors. A 1942 review praised the Hanover scholars' work, contrasting their affirmation of a hazard with the "reluctance" of English and American scientists to admit a danger. Nordmann himself noted that the head of Germany's Asbestosis Committee—Ernst Baader—was convinced of the reality of the cancer threat. The first textbook affirming the hazard was published in 1939.

In 1943, the Nazi government became the first to recognize asbestos-induced mesothelioma and lung cancer as compensable occupational diseases. U.S. attorneys would later use this Nazi-era research to prove that knowledge of an asbestos-cancer link pre-dated the time when Johns-Manville and other asbestos producers claimed they first could have known about the hazard. German experts in occupational medicine—even those in in major industries like I.G. Farben--had recognized the cancer hazard by the early 1940s.[12]

Why, then, did it take so long, outside Germany, for the lung cancer-asbestos link to be taken seriously? What we have to reckon with is both the conservatism built into postwar epidemiology and the postwar political disregard for all things German, the stigma of Nazism. The latter point is fairly straightforward; as Philip Enterline suggests in his history of asbestos cancer: "German literature and German laws were not very popular in 1943," and for some time thereafter.

The epidemiologic point, however, is more subtle. To begin with, the science of epidemiology as developed in the 1950s required large numbers of "cases"—which were not always available to early asbestos researchers. Even after Nordmann's 1938 study, the sum total of *all* the world's known asbestos cancers was only six (Nordmann had added two new cases). Epidemiologists were not impressed. As late as 1956, American epidemiologists could claim there were "too few cases and too little epidemiologic data to establish a significant relationship" between lung cancer and asbestos. The difficulty was not just industrial obstinacy or epidemiologic myopia or distrust of German science; the difficulty was also in the new methods of obtaining scientific proof. The German scholars who had claimed to have established the link relied not on epidemiology but on clinical and pathological insights. Clinicians examining patients and pathologists examining corpses had noticed asbestotics coming down with the disease, but also that lung cancers were most often found in those parts of the lungs where the inhaled fibers tended to concentrate (especially the lower lobes). Detailed study of individual cases was sufficient, for these early scholars, to generate reliable conclusions about causality.

Postwar epidemiologists and biostatisticians set little store by evidence of this sort. (Richard Doll in the 1990s ridiculed Nordmann's claim to have "proven" the asbestos-cancer link by examining only two individual cases.)[13] The "higher" standard of proof required by the new field of epidemiology prejudiced scholars against the insights gained through clinical investigations, a loss Christopher Sellers has characterized as "the vanishing clinician's eye."[14] The net effect in the field of cancer research was to slow recognition of the asbestos hazard: the consensus achieved in Germany in the early 1940s would not obtain in Britain or the United States until many years later. Science and political stigma thus conspired—at least for a time—to confine the truth to shadows.

Chemical Industry Cancers

Nazi medical interests in chemical industry cancers were often contradictory. Many health officials appear to have been genuinely worried about occupational health, but the rapid buildup of the arms industry and the single-minded focus on production eventually shifted attention away from cancer hazards. Efforts to eliminate illness turned into efforts to eliminate sick workers from the factory, from the hospital, and in certain cases from life itself. The war on disease turned into a war on the diseased. As one prominent Nazi doctor put it after the war: Nazi physicians wanted "to eliminate sickness by eliminating the sick."[15] I.G. Farben's Auschwitz plant put this into practice by never allowing more than five percent of its total work-force to be hospitalized at any given time. When the five percent figure was exceeded, camp physicians performed a selection, and the unfortunate selectees were sent to Birkenau and gassed.

German fascists wanted healthy workers, but they also wanted a peaceful and productive atmosphere on the shop floor. Factory health precautions often required expensive equipment redesign, or time-consuming changes in the production process. Especially during the war, labor officials were often reluctant to point to chronic hazards. And cancers became less and less of a concern as the war dragged on: the 1944 volume of the journal *Arbeitsmedizin*, for example, discussed how and what workers should eat at great length, but made no mention of cancer.

The constitutionalist bias of "Selection medicine" also meant that when, say, occupational bladder cancer was discussed, this was often in the context of how to weed out workers judged particularly "vulnerable" to the disease. Industrial hygienists prior even to 1933 seized on the idea of differential vulnerability: In 1930 and 1932, the head physician of I.G. Farben's Institute for the Research and Treatment of Occupational Diseases argued that genealogical studies should be conducted to determine which among a pool of candidate workers were more likely to have "tumor predispositions" to allow a "more appropriate selection" of workers for hazardous positions. After 1933, with the new premium on genetic determinism, such proposals became more common. Franz Koelsch, perhaps the most highly-regarded occupational physician of the era, tried to identify certain "constitutional types" that would be more appropriate for work in the steel industry, others that would work well in the chemical industry, and so forth. A great deal of effort went into finding ways to identify resistant workers, under the name of "Selection Medicine." This helps us understand even Hueper's ideas, expressed into the late 1950s, that Negroes were more appropriate for certain kinds of jobs, given their resistance to certain skin ailments.

In Germany, the idea of barring "cancer-sensitive" workers from jobs involving exposure to chemical hazards was eventually sidelined by the more radical prospect of using "enemies of the state" to do the dirtiest jobs. Hundreds of thousands of slave and foreign workers were brought to Germany to service German factories during the war; at I.G. Farben alone, an estimated 63,000 foreign workers, 10,000 concentration camp prisoners, and 10,000 prisoners of war were forced onto factory floors. Thousands of prisoners worked at other facilities--the secret underground bomb factory near Nordhausen, for example, where radioactive nuclear waste was fashioned into radiological weapons. Many of these men and women must have developed cancers, but records have simply not been kept. Cancer may have been the least of their concerns, since many succumbed to the regime's policy of "destruction through work."

The social policies ultimately favored by the government equated value of life with ability to work. When policy-makers eventually decided to kill the mentally ill and physically handicapped in German hospitals, many of those patients capable of productive work were spared. The goal of occupational medicine likewise became a worker who would remain productive until retirement and then pass away shortly thereafter. As Hermann Hebestreit of the German Labor Front put the matter: the aim was to reduce the difference between the age of retirement and the age of death—ideally to zero. Werner Bockhacker, chief of the DAF's health office, put forward pretty much the same idea. In the idealized Nazi scheme of things, workers would work long and hard and then die—saving for the *Volksgemeinschaft* the financial burdens of the elderly and "unproductive" infirm.

Certain aspects of this, of course, can be regarded as a continuation of pre-Nazi policies. Germany's state-supported social insurance system long pre-dated the Nazi era: the "sickness funds" established in 1883 gave the state a strong interest in reducing medical costs, which turned out to be a key factor in the Nazi "euthanasia operation" to rid the Reich of "useless eaters."

What was new in the Nazi era was this ideology of an all-pervasive, medico-utopian, legally-sanctioned racial supremacy. Racial supremacy was crucial also for the use of prisoners of war as "subjects" in concentration camp experiments—many of which can be viewed as efforts to enlarge the field of occupational health and safety. The freezing and low-pressure experiments conducted at Dachau, for example, were designed to advance the field of flight physiology, providing the knowledge-base needed to rescue pilots exposed to icy cold air or water or the rapid decompression associated with high-altitude bailouts (Figure 7). Military authorities wanted to know whether a pilot downed in the North Sea and exposed to water at a temperature of, say, ten degrees Celsius for three hours might still be alive and worth a rescue effort. Many of the most notorious experiments were designed to answer practical questions of this sort.

Germany, in effect, had two systems of occupational health and safety: one for the racially desirable and one for the racially inferior. The five million forced laborers brought into Germany to work in factories rarely benefited from safeguards. Even for "healthy" Germans, protections were weakened from the permanent state of emergency and political terror. Shirking in this climate became tantamount to treason, inability to work a virtual death sentence.

It is in this context that the "progressive" measures of occupational medicine in the Third Reich must be situated. Nazi leaders in certain instances took steps to protect workers health and safety, though not everyone was equal when it came to obtaining help. Inability to work could itself become a death sentence, especially if there were doubts about your "racial fitness." Many aspects of the Nazi efforts to improve health were ultimately as cynical as all those signs in iron in the gateways to concentration camps, reassuring the deported that work would make you free.

Notes

[1] Certain parts of this presentation draw from Robert Procter. *Nazi War on Cancer*. Princeton: Princeton University Press, 1999.

[2] *Trials of War Criminals before the Nuernberg Military Tribunals*. Washington D.C.: U.S. Government Printing Office, 1953, vol. 1, p. 721.

[3] Ibid., p. 720

[4] Wilhelm Engelmann, "The Present Position of Radium Emanation Therapy in Germany," *British Journal for Physical Medicine*, N.S. 1 (1938): 229-30 & 244.

[5] Gerhard Kahlau and A. Schraub, "Krebserzeugung durch Strahlung, insbesondere Schneeberger Lungenkrebs" in: Boris Rajewsky and Michael Schön, eds. *Biophysics*: Part I. Wiesbaden, Germany: Office of the Military Government, 1948, pp. 132-66.

[6] Proctor op. cit., pp. 186-92.

[7] Hans Krebs to Heinrich Himmler, Nov. 19, 1938, and Himmler to Krebs, Dec. 15, 1938, T-175 #87, folder 193, Captured German Documents, National Archives.

[8] Jonathan E. Helmreich, *Gathering Rare Ores: The Diplomacy of Uranium Acquisition, 1943-1954*. Princeton: Princeton University Press, 1986, p. 248.

[9] Martin Nordmann, "Der Berufskrebs der Asbestarbeiter," *Zeitschrift für Krebsforschung*, 47 (1938): 288-302; Franz Koelsch, "Lungenkrebs und Beruf," *Acta Unio Internationalis Contra Cancrum*, 3 (1938): 243-51; Friedrich Hornig, "Klinische Betrachtungen zur Frage des Berufskrebses der Asbestarbeiter," *Zeitschrift für Krebsforschung*, 47 (1938): 281-87; Ludwig Teleky, "Beruflicher Lungenkrebs," *Actio Unio Internationalis Contra Cancrum* 3 (1938):253-73.

[10] Reichsarbeitsblatt, III (1940): 263. The "Richtlinien für die Bekämpfung

der Staubgefahr in Asbest verarbeitenden Betrieben" are also discussed in Ehrhardt, "Der heutige Stand," pp. 191-93.

[11] Hans-Wilfrid Wedler, *Klinik der Lungenasbestos*. Leipzig: Georg Thieme, 1939, p. 68.

[12] Eberhard Gross, "Das Carcinom vom Standpunkt des Gewerbetoxikologen," in *Chemie und Krebs*, ed. Adolf Butenandt, et al. Berlin: Chemie, 1940, pp. 101-02.

[13] Richard Doll, personal communication.

[14] Christopher Sellers, "Discovering Environmental Cancer: Wilhelm Hueper, Post-World War II Epidemiology, and the Vanishing Clinician's Eye" *Am J Public Health* 87 (1997): 1824-35.

[15] Oswald Bumke, *Erinnerungen und Betrachtungen: Der Weg eines deutschen Psychiaters*. Munich: Pflaum, 1952, p. 145.

Table: Occupational Health Journals in NS-Era (a selection)

Arbeitsmedizin: Abhandlungen über Berufskrankheiten
Arbeitsphysiologie
Arbeitsschutz
Archiv für Gewerbepathologie und Gewerbehygiene
Die Gasmaske (Auergesellschaft of Berlin)
Gesundheitsingenieur
Monatsschrift für Unfallheilkunde
Staub
Zentralblatt für Gewerbehygiene und Unfallverhütung

Comment

Occupational Health under Fascism in Italy

Carnevale F, Local Health Unit of Florence, Florence, Italy

Preamble

The study of workers' conditions under Fascism must deal with difficulties in finding adequate documentation, partly destroyed by the regime itself. There is also a lack of observers and truthful information, and "propaganda" prevails on news. Complaints and descriptions by "anti-fascists" are often incomplete and poorly documented. Consequently it's necessary to refer to the large amounts of medical journals' articles and to proceedings of medical congresses in order to indirectly describe the working conditions even if this source is ambiguous in describing the situation.

Fascism makes its entry into history by destroying the workers' parties and unions, and from that moment it integrates capitalist offensive. The condition of the working class in Fascist Regime are generally too complex to be defined uniquely.

During interwar period there has been a profound transformation of Italian society animated by a split between technical development and material life (which has mainly affected certain privileged social classes) and the overall social and civic growth of the country. The effects of modernization (which is not completed at the end of Fascism) on health is characterized by inequality and dualism, bureaucratic inefficiency, duplication and waste, excesses and deficiencies, obtuse and fiscal limitations, rhetoric of form and humiliation.

The questions Proctor asked in his seminal book *The Nazi war on cancer* can be answered in Italian case-study.

During the Fascist period medical scientists produced relevant scientific results especially in the field of clinic occupational medicine, for acute, subacute poisonings. This was mainly the result of clinical observations, rather than epidemiological or laboratory and experimental studies. Doctors could observe ill workers in hospital guards or departments and since 1934 as insurance doctors. These observations were presented at the periodical international congresses as in Budapest 1928 and Berlin 1938.

After "Liberation" the first historiography, strongly influenced by Marxism, actually overlooked some positive effects (even for health of workers) of the fascist "authoritarian modernization," because of concern to highlight, recognize the positive aspects of Fascism. Such effects were later emphasized by "revisionist" historians in 70s-80s of the twentieth century, namely by Renzo De Felice in his in-depth studies on Fascism.

With respect to technical solutions that makes it more secure jobs, occupational medicine didn't lead other countries. Even research results obtained in the Nazi allied Germany at the same time were scarcely introduced in Italy. Adoption of oppressive, primitive and uncritical "Scientific Management" was widespread. No attempt was made to introduce Human Relation approach. The principles of occupational psychology, well known in Italy thanks to father Agostino Gemelli's laboratory in Milan, was applied only to very narrow categories of workers like aircraft pilots and army members. In general the main attitude was to blame as responsible for their own safety at work the workers themselves who had no adequate knowledge and rights.

Fascism didn't take any preventive measures, precautions, based on data less conclusive than those relied on in those years and later by other countries or international bodies like ILO. Even in field of special interest for the racist policy of Fascism, like the protection of maternity and youth, no more advanced legislation was adopted to protect health and safety at work.

In substance there wasn't a "double standard" to give priority to "higher beings" than other subjects considered "inferior." Fascism did not need any inferior "race" to find a mass of workers that could be unlimitedly exploited: it just took decisions based on the social class. Germanic ally adopted this "inferior races" policy also against Italian workers recruited in various ways even by force to work in German companies during the wartime. Only the puppet government of the so-called "Repubblica di Salò" (1943-1945) adopted the same attitude of the Nazi racism, discriminating over Jews and political opponents.

The case studies of Proctor

In our country the debate about the safety of ionized radiation, radio therapy was not comprehensive and transparent. No crisis was apparent in this field.

In Italy uranium was never mined.

No report described chronic arsenic diseases.

Chromium was frequently associated in case-reports with nasal perforation and dermatological lesions.

With regard to silicosis, till the end of thirties no intervention was introduced and a false reassurance that Italian workers were not exposed was widespread. In 1938 a crisis erupted when a number of foundry workers were sacked from their work because of disease and then they claimed the liability of their employers in justice courts. In 1943 the recognition of silicosis as compensated professional disease solved the crisis. This evolution emphasized the insurance role instead of technical prevention.

In contrast to the widespread use of chrysotile especially from Balangero quarry, but also of imported crocidolite in Italy, major initiatives to protect workers from dusts were absent. No specific legislation was adopted. A lot of information were collected by Enrico Vigliani in 1940's on hygienic condition in northern Italy asbestos factories. Debate on carcinogenicity of asbestos was practically absent, differently from the allied Nazis Germany.

The growing chemical industry only in retrospect, after the onset of epidemics of cancer, clinically well-documented, took preventive actions. Paradigmatic is the case of benzene and Aromatic Amines in dye industries. Even in these cases Vigliani described the situation in a series of scientific papers.

Witnesses

> "In the Fascist system the workers are no longer 'exploited' according to a old terminology, but 'collaborators', 'producers', whose standard of life must be raised materially and morally, in relation to time and opportunities." *(Mussolini, at gathering of industrialists, 1928)*

> "Today, shivering in the twilight of life, with Fascism we heated in the bright sunshine of a youth that scored an hour of pride and faith in the meridian of History that comes us back to the glories of Imperial Rome, Rome dominator of Peoples."
> *(Gabbi, Congress of Occupational Medicine, 1928)*

> "Forcing the Italian worker to provide automatic and monotonous tasks means to sterilize the wits, make it subject to overexploitation of their forc-

es, it means to undermine the physical integrity of our race which the fascist government devotes most loving care to, because the future of Italy rests mainly on the integrity of it."
(Il Lavoro Fascista, Trade Unions Journal, 1929)

"'Undoubtedly work as a disease is a painful exception that's going away and that affects no more but the frail or stubborn people, or predisposed or scruffy,' so the doctor, in the case of lead poisoning, was right in saying to worker: 'But You just wanted to own you! Did you come just for creating a day and a little for now, by dint of negligence, neglect, lack of discipline!"
(Fambri, Director of Fascist Institute of Social Medicine, 1931)

"Our Duce, in strict compliance to the discipline of our Regime, to the Duty and to the Country, we do not believe to deserve such unfair salary reductions, we are veterans of the Homeland Battle and now we work in chemical departments of a factory (many difficult and painful for the effects of acid) in order to supply food for our children "Balilla". These industrialists gentlemen with the excuse of industrial crises take advantage of too. For them there is no decree laws, there is no 'Chart of Labor', apologizing that they can not go on, but stretching all the years the departments and they tighten our belt every fortnight. Excellency, we reported these events from 1 August onwards, approximately six hundred pounds to a head ... For us there is no one in support and so we cannot go anymore. Well, we hope to what lies ahead: God will give new blessing to our Duce, the Regime, the Homeland. Happy Easter to all"
(Spinners of Forlì Viscosa factory, 1931)

"The worker is ultimately always in the hands of factory's direction and does not approach the unions to explain his demands because company can sack them immediately under the most different causes and without the unions are able to change the measures. It is said that the management of establishments organized his security service entrusted to private guards, that lives in and outside the establishments is controlled so much as to cause amongst the mass a feeling of permanent concern ..."
(Report of an informant sent from the political police to investigate about the Marzotto company, 1936)

"The fight against silicosis, as against other work diseases is a struggle for the improvement of the race: fast solution of this problem through mandatory reporting of silicosis as occupational disease for the moment, is the duty of doctors and Fascists aware of the ethical responsibility that have taken, besides the pride of belonging to a State which in matters of Social Security is second to no other country in the world."
(Quarelli, Congress of Occupational Medicine, 1938)

Sources

Annali della Fondazione GG Feltrinelli, *La classe operaia durante il fascismo.* Milano: Feltrinelli; 1981.

Carnevale F, Baldasseroni A, *Mal da lavoro. Storia della salute dei lavoratori.* Roma-Bari: Laterza; 1999.

De Felice R, *Mussolini il fascista, L'organizzazione dello Stato fascista, 1925-1929.* Torino: Einaudi; 1969.

De Felice R, *Mussolini il duce, Lo Stato totalitario, 1936-1940.* Torino: Einaudi; 1981.

Proctor RN, *La Guerra di Hitler al cancro.* Milano: Raffaello Cortina Editore; 2000. [original ed. Proctor RN, *The Nazi war on cancer.* Princeton; Princeton University Press: 1999.]

Comment

Occupational Health in Japan During the "15 years war"

Bernard Thomann
Institut National des Langues et Civilisations Orientales
Paris, France

From the beginning of the 20th century, foreign influences were strong on Japanese occupational medicine. German industrial hygienism was the first to reach Japan. Gotô Shimpei, a civil servant, introduced Industrial hygienism in Japan after having defended a doctor thesis in the University of Munich in 1893. By his role in the hygiene bureau of the Home Ministry and his publication on the textile workers tuberculosis,[1] he was one of the main initiator of the debate that ended in the vote of a Factory law in 1911 (enacted in 1916). This factory law had for main purpose to regulate the working conditions of children and women, to create a factory inspector corps and to introduce compensation for work accident and industrial diseases. After World war one, German influence reached Japan through social hygiene and industrial physiology. The director of the first research center on occupational diseases (Research center on labor science, *Rôdô kagaku kenkyûjo*), Teruoka Gitô, studied physiology at the University of Berlin with Max Rubner and social hygiene with Albert Grotjahn.

German influence was not alone. The safety first movement was introduced in Japan from the United States during the 1910s, but it became particularly influent after world war 1, with safety weeks and safety days regularly taking place. It became a tool for the promotion of class cooperation in the hand of the Association of industrial welfare (*Sangyô fukuri kyôkai*), an association close to the Home Ministry. Recognition of industrial diseases made a great step forward thanks to Japan's ILO membership during in the interwar period. Indeed, Japan ratified the 1925 Convention on industrial diseases in 1928, and the 1934 Convention in 1936. For example, Silicosis was recognized as an Industrial disease in 1930.

However, from the 1930s, there was a growing Nazi influence on Japanese occupational health. Social hygiene tended to mutate in racial hygiene. In the books of Teruoka Gitô, there was already mention of racial hygiene at the end of the 1920's, however, from the middle of the 1930, under the influence of the Nazis, this trend became stronger. References to authors such as Max von Gruber, Ignaz Kaup, or Fritz Lenz became dominant and reference to eugenism (such notion as degeneration- *taika-entartung*) became more numerous.[2] In 1940, a national Eugenic law was voted.

After the beginning of the war with China in 1937, mobilization of the working force became a priority. The German *Deutsche arbeitfront* became an example and, in 1938, the Japanese Industrial patriotic association (*Sangyô hôkokukai*) was created for purpose of spiritual mobilization and collaboration between workers and employers. Occupational health was also integrated as the Research center for labor science became part of the *Sangyô hôkokukai* in 1941. Spiritual mobilization and mental fitness of the workers became a quasi obsession with the beginning of the war. Expert in the occupational field became persuaded that working culture, contaminated by socialism had to be changed. For example the word "workers" "*rôdôsha*" was not used anymore because it was also used by labor unions and Marxists and was replaced by alternative words to designate the industrial laborers such as *sangyô rômusha* , *kinrôsha*, *sangyô senshi*, *sangyô jûgyôin*. The German movement *Kraft durch freude* had also a certain influence in that to crate this new culture all kind of cultural activity were organized from musical activities to calligraphy.[3]

War mobilization from 1937 had obviously a very negative impact on industrial health as there was an extensive use of slave labor from China and Korea. Indeed, more than 600 000 Koreans were forced to work in Japanese industry. 300,000 Koreans were used in Japanese mines between 1939 and 1945, more than one third of all miners. 38,935 Chinese aged from 11 years old to 78 years were moved in Japan to work in 135 mines, docks and constructions sites. According to a 1946 survey, there had in those camps, 6,830 deaths, a mortality rate of 17.5 percent.[4] There was also an increasing use of female workers and a weakening of legal protection in the field of labor condition. From October 1940 until February 1944, the number of men working for manufacturing industry decreased from 6,18 to 4,74 millions and the number of women increased from 1,95 to 2,25 millions. This growing need of female labor was the source of tension inside the government, between the Ministry of Industry and the Ministry of Ammunition, on one hand, whose priority was an increase of the industrial production, and, on the other hand, the Ministry of Welfare, created in 1938, which had a pro birth policy, and had for priority the preservation of the quality of the population and the amelioration of the workers physical condition. As the result, there was on the one hand a special emphasis on monitoring workers health more closely. From 1938, enterprises of 500 employees (100 employees from 1940) and more, had the obligation to have a factory doctor who had to inspect the factory once a year. From 1940, enterprises had the obligation to conduct medical check-up at the time of the hiring and one or twice a year, and to keep the workers medical record for at least three years. However, there was also, one the other hand, a weakening of the legal protection. For example, in 1943, the Special edict on factories in wartime eliminated all the interdictions concerning female labor in dangerous place and between 10 o'clock in the evening and 4 o'clock in the morning.[5]

Wartime Japan is not only a time of deterioration in the occupational health situation, but also of changing priorities. For example, researcher of the Research center for labor sciences or the Japanese association of industrial hygiene, the main association of companies doctor, tended to ignore industrial diseases, such as silicosis, that had the priority during the 1920s and the first half of the 1930s, mainly because of the influence of the ILO and the growing social movement, and started to focus on health questions more directly linked to the living conditions of the war and the need to increase the production. Because of the deterioration of working and living condition of female workers, tuberculosis was an especially acute problem. In certain industries such as the food industry, the rate of incidence, according the health insurance statistics, was of more than 70 for thousand, and this rate increased rapidly in all industries.[6] The coincidence between the emphasis on physical condition and the food shortage, made the question of nutrition very acute. Based on the family budget surveys and research in dietetics, expert tried to calculate the minimum salary needed to keep a worker and his family in good health. During the war there was an increase in the work accident rate that had an influence on the productivity. Safety weeks became part of the mobilization policy for total war as the safety first movement also made campaigns for the protection during air raid which became very numerous from the beginning of 1943. During the war, the Research center for labor sciences *(Nihon rôdô kagaku kenkyûjo)* grew bigger and made emphasis on those new priorities. It also started large research on subject not directly linked to industrial work. It made for example a very large survey in 1939, on the way to adapt better the lifestyle of Japanese settlers with very tough climate of Manchuria.[7]

We can conclude that Japanese industrial health policies presented during World War Two, very common patterns with the German case, in particular, ideological patterns such as the reject of class struggle or the mobilization for total war. But the Japanese case had also particularities such a discourse very much based on spiritual mobilization around the emperor that didn't suppress but kind of attenuated biological and eugenic discourses

Notes

[1] Gotô S. *Shokugyô eiseihô. Dai Nippon shiritsu eiseikai zasshi.* 1888-1889; 63-68.

[2] Teruoka G. *Shaikai eiseigaku.* Tôkyô: Tohôdô; 1935.

[3] Yanagizawa O. *Senzen senki Nihon no keizaishisô to nachizumu.* Tôkyô: Iwanami shoten; 2008. p. 227-242.

[4] Underwood W. Chinese Forced Labor, the Japanese Government and the Prospects for Redress, Japan Focus [Internet]. 2005 July. Available from: http://www.japanfocus.org/-William-Underwood/1693

[5] Miura T. *Rôdô to kenkô no rekishi* (vol. 4). Kawasaki: Rôdô kagaku kenkyûjo; 1981.

[6] Rôdô kagaku. 1941; 8: 59-88.

[7] Miura T. *Teruoka Gitô: Rôdôkagaku o tsukutta otoko*, Tôkyô, Ripuropôto; 1991.

Comment

Occupational Health in the First Francoism, 1939-1953

Alfredo Menéndez-Navarro
Department of History of Science, University of Granada
Granada, Spain

The role of Occupational Health in a destroyed and isolated country

In comparison to Nazi Germany and Fascist Italy, the so-called First Francoism (1939-1953) presents a quite different setting. The regime emerged after a long and devastating civil war (1936-39); and the First Francoism was therefore a period of economic stagnation and hardship, within a context of autarchic protectionism and international isolation of the regime. Furthermore, health conditions in Spain considerably worsened by the end of the war. The destruction of health facilities, the spread of malnutrition, and outbreaks of smallpox, diphtheria, typhus and malaria epidemics shaped the health landscape in the 1940s. Infectious diseases continued to be the first cause of mortality in Spain until 1953, just one year after rationing ended.

For my overview of the relationship between occupational health and fascism in Franco's Spain, I would like to make four previous considerations. First, the violent and massive political repression during and in the aftermath of the Civil War made it necessary for Franco's regime to seek devices for its legitimization among the popular classes. Social policies became crucial to the furtherance of these aims and were adopted by the fascist party from the very beginning. Thus, healthcare and public and occupational health were mainly conceived of as instruments for political proselytism. According to fascist ideas, the aim of public health was not only the production and reproduction of the workforce, a matter of mere economics, but also, and mainly, an attempt to reintegrate the worker into the "metaphysical reality of the nation."[1]

Second, the so-called National Syndicalist Revolution, inspired by Mussolini's Italy, intended to eliminate class struggle by establishing a totalitarian society made up of totalitarian families, totalitarian municipal governments and totalitarian worker-employer unions, the so-called vertical unions. In fact, it meant that workers were deprived of the right to independent association, and their class-based unions were banned. The harsh restriction of workers' freedoms deprived them of any possible involvement in negotiating their working conditions, ensuring their subordination.[2]

Third, as in other totalitarian regimes, racial theories became a key issue in the legitimization of the new state and an instrument to explain social inequalities and justify social hierarchies (rather than social classes). However, the concept of race had a sociological rather than biological inspiration, signifying a sense of a spiritual community united by aspects such as language, culture and moral and religious factors. Eugenics in Franco's Spain needed to reconcile racial hygiene with the requirements of Catholic moral doctrine, opposed to state-imposed measures of eugenic restriction.[3]

Fourth, as in other European countries, the passing of legislation on workers' compensation at the beginning of the 20th century shaped the development and direction of Spanish Occupational Medicine. This legislation favored a compensatory approach to industrial hazards rather than an effective policy of prevention and fostered the concept of occupational medicine as "Accident Medicine," dominated by clinical concerns. Thus, the main tasks of this new specialist were the provision of efficient first aid care, the carrying out of initial and regular medical examinations, and the forensic evaluation of workers' residual capacity. This restricted vision of occupational health widened during the Republican years (1931-36), paralleling an intense period of moderate social reformism following International Labor Organization guidelines. The scope of training in occupational health widened to include the Physiology of Work, Professional Guidance, Scientific Organization of Work, Hygiene, and Work Diseases, as well as Work Accidents. However, the outbreak of the war brought this expanded vision to an end.[4]

Franco's Spain Occupational Health Scheme

The general principles of the regime's social policy were embedded in the Labor Charter proclaimed in 1938. Inspired by the Italian Fascist Carta del Lavoro (1927), the Charter legitimized the state control of labor relations on the grounds of the defense of workers and the search for national prosperity and social harmony.

The central institution of the new occupational health organization was the National Institute for Medicine and Safety at Work, set up in 1944. It was responsible for research, professional training, healthcare assistance, and rehabilitation and public health campaigns. The professional core of the new occupational health scheme was the so-called Factory Doctor. Factory Medicine was defined as «applied» Industrial Medicine and was acclaimed by its supporters as a genuine Spanish alternative for the provision of specialized care and expertise at the workplace, after the exclusion of occupational health from the remit of the newly established National Health Insurance system. Factory Doctors received an intensive six-month training course, which was mainly theoretical. The main preventive legislation was embodied in the General Regulations of Health and Safety (issued in 1940). However, its weak recommendations and the lack of compliance failed to reduce the steady rise in work accidents and occupational diseases, notably silicosis.

What were the main flaws of this scheme? Various factors contributed to its failure, including the rise of a culture of submission rather than collaboration derived from the granting of leading positions to Franco's followers in academic and public administrations. Other hindering factors included the reluctance of employers to implement the scheme, its weak supervision by the Work Inspectorate and the lack of Governmental will to enforce it. Furthermore, the lack of autonomy and inadequate training of Factory Doctors (including a poor regulation of their appointments, salary and working conditions) made them second-class medical specialists who were wholly dependent on the factory owners.

Eventually, in 1956, the establishment of a Factory Medical Service became compulsory for companies employing more than 500 workers, later extended to those employing more than 100. Nevertheless, the slow and limited implementation of the Factory Medical Services meant that most factories and workers were not even covered by the scheme. In 1969, only one in five (21.5%) of the 8.5 million insured workers were employed in factories with these services.

The main effects of the institutionalization of occupational medicine in Franco's Spain were in the clinical domain. The hospital attached to the National Institute became a seed bed for traumatology, orthopedics, and neurosurgery. In contrast, there was a very limited research agenda. The main areas investigated were lead poisoning, silicosis, industrial dermatoses, and accident surgery. There were no studies of work physiology, and a thorough review of the official journal of the Institute, launched in 1952 (*Medicina y*

Seguridad del Trabajo), confirmed that common industrial conditions like asbestosis or occupational cancer were not considered major issues. In fact, cancer did not re-emerge as a health concern in Spain until the early 1950s, when the general health conditions of the population had recovered from the harsh post-war years.[5]

The compensatory approach to occupational health

The flaws of Francoist occupational health system and its poor performance in the preventive domain seem even more evident when compare with the effectiveness of the extension of social and health insurance. This was perceived as the crux of the fascist regime's strategy to cope with industrial health and was used as a formidable propaganda tool to represent the regime as a providing and magnanimous state.

Apart from work accidents, silicosis was the main concern of this compensatory model. Dust-related diseases became a key issue in the political agenda of the regime in the 1940s. This was mainly due to the strategic role played by coal mining in the Spanish economy under the autarchic system, when almost nine-tenths of Spain's energy consumption was coal-based. In 1941, the Labor Department launched the Silicosis Scheme, a compulsory insurance scheme entirely funded by employers. The application of strict criteria during the 1940s minimized the number of silicotics approved for compensation under the scheme. Nevertheless, after the mid-1940s, workers took advantage of Francoist labor institutions to defend their interests, particularly the so-called labor tribunals. Almost 300,000 lawsuits came before these tribunals in the late 1940s. Disputes over compensation for silicosis and accidents became some of the most frequent causes.

Besides compensation and medical monitoring, very little action was taken on dust suppression during the 1940s and the 1950s, because the Scheme did not include the regulation of safety standards, and coalmining employers failed to take voluntary action to address the dust problem. By the late 1950s, the shortcomings of the dust control policy were evident even to the officials, usually reluctant to engage in any kind of public criticism of the regime. The number of pneumoconiosis sufferers receiving compensation grew steadily during the 1950s. Only the growing economic burden that compensation placed on coal companies forced a change in preventive policies during the 1960s, giving place to a new approach to the dust problem that was focused on technical prevention.[6]

ACKNOWLEDGEMENTS

This research was supported by the Spanish Ministry of Science Project HAR2009-07543.

NOTES

[1] Jiménez Lucena I. Medicina social, racismo y discurso de la desigualdad en el primer franquismo. In: Huertas R, Ortiz C, editors. *Ciencia y Fascismo*. Madrid: Doce Calles; 1998. p. 111-126.

[2] Molinero C, Ysàs P. Workers and Dictatorship: industrial growth, social control and labour protest under the Franco regime, 1939-76. In: Smith A, editor. *Red Barcelona. Social protest and labour mobilization in the twentieth century*. London: Routledge; 2002. p. 185-205.

[3] Bandrés J, Llavona R. *Psychology in Franco's concentration camps*. Psychol. Spain. 1997;1:3-9.

[4] Menéndez-Navarro A, Rodríguez-Ocaña E. From 'Accident Medicine' to 'Factory Medicine': Spanish Occupational Medicine in the Twentieth Century. In: Grieco A, Fano D, Carter T, Iavicoli S, editors. *Origins of Occupational Health Associations in the World*. Amsterdam: Elsevier Science B.V.; 2003. p. 207-216.

[5] Rodríguez-Ocaña E, Ortiz-Gómez T. Medical research in Franco's Spain. An overview. In: Presas i Puig A, editor. *Science, Scientist and Totalitarian Systems: Spanish Science during Francoism*. Berlin: Max Planck Institute for the History of Science Preprint Reihe. Forthcoming 2011

[6] Menéndez-Navarro A. The politics of silicosis in interwar Spain: Republican and Francoist approaches to occupational health. *Dynamis*. 2008; 28: 77-102.

Expanded Abstracts

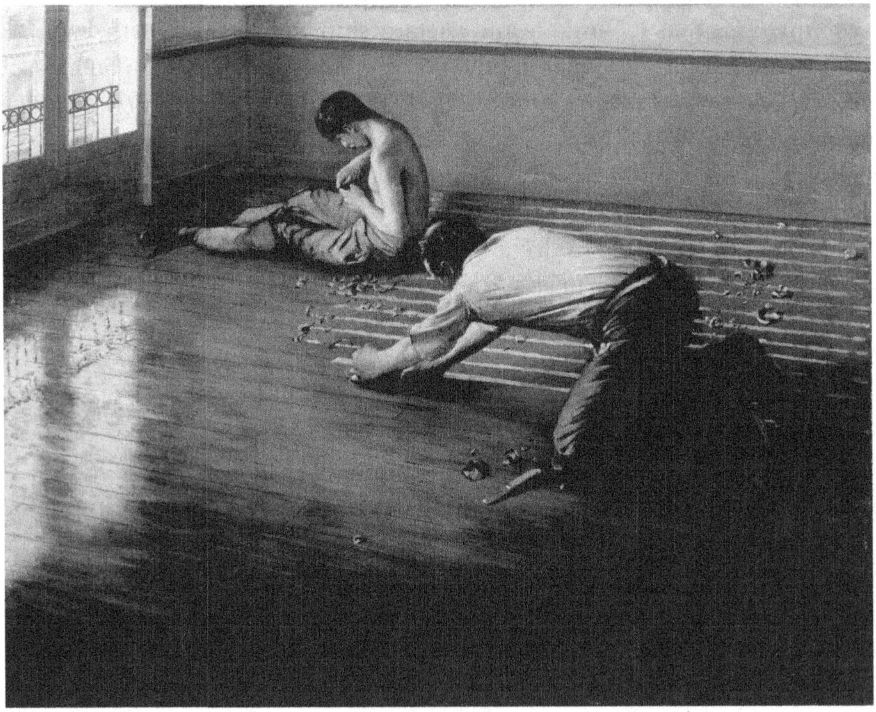

Floor scrapers: Caillebotte "Etude pour les Raboteurs de parquet." Private collection - courtesy Comité Caillebotte, Paris. 1876. Oil on canvas, 80 x 100 cm. Used with permission.

Occupational Health in Hippocratic writings

Vuorinen H. S. & Hannu T. J.
Hjelt Institute, Department of Public Health, University of Helsinki, Helsinki, Finland

Environmental health can easily trace its origin back to the Hippocratic times. A celebrated example of geographical or meteorological medicine is the famous treatise Airs, Waters, Places, which an unknown Greek physician wrote in the second half of the fifth century BC. Ideas expressed in this Hippocratic writing had a definite influence during antiquity and later (Jouanna 1999: 356, 361, 375, 478).

The history of occupational health during antiquity has received much less attention among modern scholars. The seven books of Epidemics offer some unique material which illustrates how Hippocratic doctors paid attention to the occupation (or trade) of their patients. These books contain altogether around 430 case histories. Books V and VII have at least 50 cases which are common for both books. Especially Books II, IV, V, VI and VII are heterogeneous collections of cases and other material, and most probably they had several authors and several dates of final composition. The books are dated to the late 5th and early 4th century BC, but some of the material in Books V and VII are somewhat later (Jouanna 1999: 388–390).

For the present study, both authors independently read the English translations in the Loeb Classical Library editions of the Hippocratic writings called Epidemics. They comprise case reports of different diseases or descriptions of symptoms related to diseases. We registered the occupations and the work relatedness of the case: ordinary disease, accident, work accident, occupational disease. One of the authors (HSV) checked the English texts against the Greek texts.

We used quite a liberal definition of a case: when it was possible to recognize an individual in the description then that was a case. A case could be only a name in a list of patients having some common symptoms, prognosis etc, or a case could be a lengthy description of symptoms from day to day. Social position was used as on approximate definition of occupation when the person was a slave or a servant.

The occupation (or social position) was expressed in 14.4% of the 430 cases. In 60 cases (14.0%) a single person was referred to and in two cases a group of people were dealt with. Information concerning the occupation or social position varied from zero in Book III to 27.2% of the cases in Book IV. The most often mentioned occupation was slave or servant, in 27 of 62 cases (43.5%); then came occupations of free members of the polis: fuller (4 references), shoemaker (4), and carpenter (3). The gender of the patient (or patients) was male in 72.1 % of the 61 cases when it was expressed together with occupation.

Four cases (Epidemics 4.20f, 5.45, 5.74 [the same in 7.36], 6.8.30) were most certainly occupational accidents and three cases (Epidemics 5.16, 5.26, 5.32) were probably occupational accidents, but other interpretations are also possible. All the accidents happened to males. Three of them were falls, one was a crush of a finger, one a needle stick injury, one a horse kick and in one case a cart rode over the victim. Two of the occupational accidents were related to harbor and/or ships. Outcome was reported in five cases: it was fatal in four cases and in only one case the person survived.

Health problems related to work were described in eight instances (Epidemics 4.25, 4.27, 4.50, 6.3.8, 6.3.9, 6.7.1[two cases], 7.122). A group of people is described in two cases (Epidemics 6.7.1). Four cases were related to musculoskeletal complaints, and the remaining four cases comprised easily tired from work, quinsy, fever, and impotence. The most illustrative description is the so called cough of Perinthus (Epidemics 6.7.1., for a discussion of the cough of Perinthus, see Grmek 1989: 305–339). Physical workload was connected to the symptoms of the "cough": slaves and those, who labored with their hands or rode horses or did more walking or other exertion, suffered more.

We found no cases of occupational diseases, when a modern definition of occupational disease is used. It has been thought that lead poisoning is described in the Epidemics (Sigerist 1945: 46). "The one from the mines: right hypocondrium stretched, spleen large, belly tight, rather hard; flatulent. He was pale. His went to the left knee. Relapse." (Epidemics 4.25) Using imagination, the symptoms described can be fitted to symptoms of lead poisoning. However, type of mining (silver or other), working with lead or any occupation or work process (e.g. melting of ore) is not mentioned. Therefore the diagnosis of lead poisoning is poorly grounded.

Interestingly, the positive effects of work were also realized in Epidemics, in sections like "Labor is food for the joints and the flesh ..." (Epidemics 6.5.4.) or "Healthy discipline, not gluttonizing, not avoiding work (Epidemics 6.4.18)."

Most of the case histories were short and deficient concerning characteristics of the patient. Usually only the gender, but occasionally also the age of the patient was mentioned. In the case histories the referred occupation is not always that of the patient. In a few cases the occupation mentioned refers to the owner of the house or slave. With these reservations we can, however, conclude that occupation (or social position) of the patient was not uncommonly noticed by the Hippocratic physician. Against the 14% of cases with occupation (or social position) mentioned in Epidemics, we may ponder: how often an occupation (or social position) is expressed in a random sample of case histories from a modern general practitioner?

Although our focus was on the seven books consisting Epidemics, there are scattered references throughout the Hippocratic writings to diseases related to the work or activities of people. Considering the occupational accidents and the work-related problems described in the Epidemics together with the evidence in the other Hippocratic writings it can be concluded that the Hippocratic doctor was well aware that health was related to work. On the base of Corpus Hippocraticum and later medical writings we may, however, conclude that in antiquity there was no place for occupational health in the modern sense of the concept.

References

Epidemics, Books I and III. In: *Hippocrates* Volume I. with an English translation by W. H. S. Jones. The Loeb Classical Library, Cambridge: Harvard University Press, 1923–2004, pp. 146–287.

Epidemics, Books II, IV-VII. In: *Hippocrates* Volume VII. Edited and translated by W.D. Smith. The Loeb Classical Library. Cambridge: Harvard University Press, 1994.

Grmek MD. *Diseases in the Ancient Greek World.* Translated by Mireille Muellner and Leonard Muellner. Baltimore & London: The Johns Hopkins University Press, 1989.

Jouanna J. *Hippocrates*. Baltimore & London: The Johns Hopkins University Press, 1999.

Sigerist HE.*Civilization and Disease*. Ithaca: Cornell University Press, 1945.

Work and Disease in Greco-Roman world: Myth and Reality

Michele A. Riva[1,2], Daniela Fano D[3], Vittorio A. Sironi[1], Giancarlo Cesana2.

[1]*Research Centre on the History of Biomedical Thought, University of Milano Bicocca, Milan, Italy*

[2]*Research Centre on the Public Health, University of Milano Bicocca, Milan, Italy*

[3]*Department of Occupational Health, "Clinica del Lavoro Luigi Devoto," University of Milan, Milan, Italy*

The descriptions of work-related hazards in Greco-Roman world are inconspicuous in ancient medical texts, where the occupation of the patient doesn't seem to be clearly considered as an aetiological element in the pathogenesis of diseases, even if it is often cited by ancient physicians in case histories. Indeed, according to Donald Hunter, the working man was neglected in ancient medical practice since the most harmful occupations were done by slaves and prisoners, whose health conditions were little considered.[1] Actually, a lot of information on the workers' condition in the classical period may be obtained by analyzing non-medical authors, such as poets, historians and politicians, who incidentally treated this subject in their writings.

According to these sources, during this period the most unhealthy and harmful work was metal mining. In particular, Lucretius (ca. 98-55 BC) claimed these workers died after brief period ("De rerum natura", VI, 813-814), as confirmed also by the poet Ovid (ca. 43 BC-17 AD) in the "Metamorphoses" (I, 138-140). Referring to Silius Italicus, the Roman poet Statius (ca. 45-96 AD) wrote that the gold miners returned all pale-faced (viso pallidus) and yellow as the metal they have unearthed ("Silvae", IV, 7, 13-16). Primitive tools - such as loose bladders, bags and sacks tied over the face - were employed to avoid inhalation of dusts, as described by Pliny the Elder (23-79 AD) and Julius Pollux (124-192 AD).[2]

Other important information on the work-related diseases in Greco-Roman world may come from satirical poets and comic playwrights, when they laughed at work-related physical defects. So, the sore eyes of sulphur workers and the varicose veins of soothsayers were targeted and ridiculed by satirists Martial ("Epigrammaton," XII, 57, 14) and Juvenal ("Satirae," 6, 397) respectively, in the first centuries of the Roman Empire.

Unlike manual workers, farmers and soldiers were highly protected during the classical period. Indeed, in ancient society the rural workers and the armed forces played an essential role in feeding and defending the population. Moreover, the war allowed recruitment of new slaves who could be used for heavy manual labour. So, it should come as no surprise that physicians were assigned to military units and in camp-based hospitals (valetudinaria) and that in time of peace those hospitals were used for the medical treatment of rural workers (slaves too). In particular, Columella (4-70 AD) first mentioned hospitals in the farms ("De Re Rustica," XI, 1, 18) and Varro (116-27 BC) claimed that farmers and slaves working in the fields were taken on by physicians, usually from a servile class ("De Re Rustica," I, 16, 4).[3]

Finally, a useful source for understanding culture and society in the Greco-Roman world may be represented by classical mythology. The euhemeristic interpretation of some myths and legends recalls suggestive hypotheses on health conditions of some ancient occupations. In particular, in the antiquity, one of the most dangerous and harmful workplace was the forge. Juvenal, talking about a smith who made swords, father of rhetorician Demosthenes, described him as sore-eyed ("Satirae," 10, 130-132) due to the workplace condition. Moreover the noise-induced hearing loss in forge hammering workers had been known since ancient times. In Greek mythology, Hephaestus, the smith of gods and heroes, worked in a forge with the Cyclopes, his assistants. Called Vulcan in Rome, he was also the most industrious of the gods (Plato referred him as the "patron" of the craftsmen; "Laws," XI, 920 D, 56) but he was also the only god who was sick. He was lame and had to walk with a stick. His son, the Argonaut bronze-smith Palaimonius was misshapen and likewise the smiths in Nordic legends (the Teutonic Wieland, the Scandinavian Volundr and the Finnish Ilmarien) were lame. In addition, in prehistoric cultures, the craftsmen were often depicted as cripples. Some scholars proposed this mythological connection between lameness and work at forge be originated by chronic arsenic poisoning and consequent neuritis of the extremities occurred in the Anatolian metallurgists of the third millennium BC, when they smelted arsenic-copper minerals and alloys or hardened with arsenic copper or brass vessels.[4] Actually, the myth itself is against this hypothesis: the Greek poet Homer stated that Hephaestus was crippled and misshapen from his birth (Odyssey, 8, 267) and this finding is in contrast to an occupational aetiology. According to Donald Hunter, these legends may suggest that "at an early stage of society the trade of a smith was regarded by common consent as suitable for a lame."[1] People with physical anomalies and unable to become soldiers, farmers or sportsmen in Olympic Games were presumably addressed towards less valued (and protected) occupations, such as the work at forge. Likewise, the work of smith was considered suitable for the Cyclops, orb-eyed giants, who would be theoretically not fit to work in a forge due to the visual problems well described by Juvenal. So, in a euhemeristic key, the legends of the lame smiths and the Cyclopes provide us precious information on the relationship between work and disease in Greco-Roman world. The physical disabilities, protected by our modern legislation, were instead considered as appropriate for manual and heavy work in a society where body beauty, harmony and athleticism were the main values.

In conclusion, in addition to medical sources, a thorough study of workers' health condition in the Greco-Roman world should also consider non-medical literature (including myths and legends) as well as cultural, economic and social issues.

For correspondence: Michele Augusto Riva, Research Centre on the History of Biomedical Thought, Centro Studi sulla Storia del Pensiero Biomedico, University of Milano Bicocca, Villa Serena, Ospedale San Gerardo di Monza, via Pergolesi 33, 20900, Monza, Italy. E-mail: michele.riva@unimib.it

References

1 Hunter D. *The Diseases of Occupations*. 5th ed. London: Engling Universities Press; 1974.
2 Rosen G. *A history of public health*. Expanded ed. Baltimore: Johns Hopkins University Press; 1993.
3 White KD. *Roman farming*. London: Thames & Hudson; 1970.
4 Nriagu JO. Occupational exposure to lead in ancient times. *Sci Total Environ*. 1983;31:105-16.

Modern Dilemmas in Occupational Medicine and Insights from the Jewish Law-Halacha: Nothing is New Under the Sun

Yehuda Lerman
Department of Epidemiology and Preventive Medicine
School of Public Health Tel- Aviv University, Tel Aviv, Israel

Introduction

Halacha, often referred to as "Hebrew or Jewish Law," is the collective body of biblical and rabbinic law regarding every aspect of life, and incorporates legal precedents from the Mishna, Talmud, and post-Talmudic literature. Halacha is vibrant with its Responsa (questions and answers), written rulings handed down throughout the ages that remain valid to this very day.

The Hypothesis

Searching Halacha can serve as a valuable research tool in tracing the history of occupational medicine.

Materials and Methods

Halachic literature shows clearly that diverse issues of modern occupational medicine were always of deep concern to Jewish communities. Presented here is a specific case of a work accident that occurred some 2000 years ago, but has been discussed ever since.

The Work Accident

This case from the Babylonian Talmud[1] describes a work accident involving a porter[2] who was hired to carry a certain specified load which the employer increased by one kab (1.3 kilograms) without his knowing, and, as a consequence, the porter collapsed.

Discussion

According to Rabbi Meir (1st Century), the employer was liable.[1] Three scholars of the Babylonian Talmud also gave opinions: Abbaye (4th century), said the additional weight struck the porter as soon as he lifted it, and he, not realizing the load was too heavy for him, collapsed under it. Rava, from the same period, explained: "You may say that it did not strike him down immediately, but this applies only with regard to extra pay. If the load exceeds the weight agreed upon by even a kab, the porter is entitled to additional remuneration." The third, Rav Ashi, head of Sura Academy, said: "The porter might have thought he had been struck by weakness," implying that although he broke under the additional weight, as a sensible person he did not drop the load, thinking that the fault lay in his own weakness, being unaware that the weight was greater than had been stipulated.

The style of the Babylonian Talmud is concise, and close attention and hard thinking are required to understand the contexts. This is where we need the commentaries of the Talmud, the most important and prominent being those of the 11th century Rashi (Rabbi Shlomo Yitzhaki), who was the author of the first comprehensive commentary of the Talmud, and considered the "father" of all Talmud and Bible commentaries.

Rashi explains[1] that according to the Talmud the weight a medium sized person can carry is 30 Kabs, and the addition of even one kab is significant, so the one who adds the weight (the employer) is liable. Since the upper limit of weight lifting was set at 30 Kabs (40 kilograms) for a medium sized person, we understand that the limit varied according to the person's size. The current NIOSH and ACGIH standards define upper limits for lifting weights at 23-32 kilograms, but do not relate to the person's size.

A search of ancient Roman Law by Prof. Emeritus Alfredo Rabbelo[3] did not uncover a similar upper limit standard value for lifting weights. In fact, it is suggested that the TLV for lifting weights described in the Talmud in the 1st and the 2nd centuries was indeed the first time that the concept of standards in occupational health was introduced.

What was the ruling regarding the porter who had to carry the additional weight? Who was liable?

Four giants of Halacha who lived during the 11th - 16th centuries concluded that the employer was liable for the work-related injury of the porter: The Rif - Rabbi Isaac al-Fasi (Algeria, Spain), the Rambam, or Maimonides (Spain, Egypt), the Rosh, or Rabbi Asher ben Jechiel (Germany, Spain), and Rabbi Yosef Karo, famous for his renowned Shulchan Aruch, which is generally regarded as the most authoritative compilation of Halacha since the Talmud itself. Rabbi Karo reasoned that "the employer was liable for the injury suffered by the porter who was laden with an additional kab in excess of the weight he was hired to carry. In spite of the fact that the porter...sensed the heavy weight of the load, he presumed this was attributable to his illness."

However the Ramban, a famous Bible and Talmud scholar expressed doubt, and questioned the liability of the employer:[1]

1. Unlike the case of hiring a boat or a camel where the renter is considered guardian of the object, in the case of an employer, he is not the guardian of the person, so there can be no grounds for damages.

2. The obligation can also not be based on the person who caused the injury since this is not directly considered a trauma.

Jewish scholars continued to refer to this accident, and an interesting issue was raised by Rabbi Natan Shapira of Poland, who agreed the employer was liable, but additionally introduced the latency period factor. He noted that if the injury occurred even after one hour or more, the employer would still be liable, pointing out that questions regarding the latency period and exposure to risk factors were raised centuries ago.

Another interesting commentary was made by Rabbi Katz of Poland who emphasized that although the standard of 30 kab or 40 kg. was the standard in the 1st and 2nd centuries but had changed over the years, the employer would always be held liable if he added a weight 3.3% of the maximum allowable.

Other comments included a response by Rabbi Hakohen of Poland (18th century), who made a clear distinction between a direct blow, and an indirect cause of an accident. Rabbi I. Z. Melzer differentiated between the weight added to the porter's load (low chance of injury), and injury from a broken machine (high chance of injury).

These principles were applied to modern Israeli Law in a recent ruling involving a bank officer who fell at the premises where renovations had been made, and claimed the injury was a direct result of negligence and lack of concern for a safe working environment. Although the defendants lay contributory blame on the plaintiff for not taking care, the judge ruled in his favor, imposing full liability on the defendants based largely on the Rav Ashi view that an employer is liable for injury caused, even for a remiss action of an employee.[4]

Summary

The Halacha is a valuable research tool for tracing the history of occupational medicine, for the ancient world had little documentary evidence regarding occupational health and disease. Halacha case studies and legal texts deal with some of the very same dilemmas that face occupational physicians today, and its rulings, rendered so very long ago, remain applicable and significant today.

Special thanks to Rabbi Udi Hadad and Prof. A. Oppenheimer for their assistance in the preparation of this manuscript. Thanks to A. Aviram for her editorial assistance.

References

1 Baba Metzia, 80b (trans. Soncino).

2 Ayali, M., *A Nomenclature of Workers and Artisans in Talmudic and Midrashic Literature*. Hakibbutz Hameuchad Publishing House; Tel Aviv, 2001.

3 Rabbelo, Alfredo (Prof. Emeritus), Personal communication, Hebrew University, Jerusalem, Israel

4 Shterenlicht, Judge Nahum, Ruling on "Roni Zadok vs. First International Bank Ltd. and Others." Tel Aviv, June 25, 2006.

5 Gochfeld, M., Chronological History of Occupational Medicine. *JOEM* 2005:47:96-114

Occupational Exposures and Transnational Networks in African Uranium Mines

Gabrielle Hecht
University of Michigan, Ann Arbor, MI, USA

The labor of African uranium miners has fueled atomic weapons and nuclear reactors around the world for over six decades, but remains invisible in histories of occupational health, the nuclear age, and Africa. The papers on which this talk was based focus on workers at the COMUF mine in Gabon and the Rössing mine in Namibia. They examine how these men understood, framed, and deployed their radiation exposures from the inception of each mine (1957 in Gabon, 1976 in Namibia) to the present. At both mines, occupational exposures were initially kept hidden from workers. By interpellating two very different sets of regional and transnational networks, however, workers at both mines were able to develop independent methods of knowledge and research production exposures became visible, material, and political. But the results of these efforts differed dramatically. In Namibia, workers found ways to conduct their own secret monitoring of health effects, and ultimately changed labor and health monitoring practices at the mine. In Gabon, former miners are seeking reparations in international courts, so far unsuccessfully. The papers argue that nuclear things in African places were produced and dissolved in frictions between the transnational politics of knowledge, the remains of colonial power, and hopes for a healthier and wealthier future. Radiation shaped workers' bodies; sometimes it also shaped their political possibilities.

How–and when–do workers, managers, doctors, or lawyers know that radiation exposure has occurred? Instruments, labor relations, scientific disciplines, expert controversy, and lay knowledge combine to create assemblages of social and technical things that make certain hazards and health effects visible, and others invisible. Assemblages exist and operate on multiple geographical scales simultaneously–local, national, transnational, global–and are shaped by politics at all these levels. Consider this question: does exposure to radon gas cause cancer? Uranium atoms decay into radon, which in turn decays into other elements known as its "daughters." These decays release radioactive alpha particles, which miners inhale. Determining causality via accepted scientific practice demands isolating the effects of radon exposure–deciding whether illness in uranium miners comes only from radon exposure, or also from other contaminants. There's also the question of deciding what constitutes a radiation effect. Lung cancer? Genetic mutations? Epidemiologists and geneticists respond differently. When do "effects" occur? Is lung cancer 30 years after the victim's last exposure an "effect"? Labor lawyers and mining corporations offer different answers.

Regardless of perspective, all these questions ultimately required knowing how much radiation mineworkers absorb. Before the 1980s, personal dosimetry–giving each worker a film badge or a dosimeter pen–only detected the external exposures produced by gamma rays emitted by radioactive rocks. Such instruments did not detect the alpha radiation emitted by inhaled radon daughters. In many places, mine managers also feared personal dosimetry would scare workers by alerting them to an otherwise invisible danger. Ambient dosimetry could accommodate the heavier instruments required to "capture" radon daughters. Less personally intrusive, it involved installing instruments throughout the mine and averaging out their readings. But averages didn't account for the experience of men assigned to "hot spots:" spots far from air intakes, where reduced ventilation meant elevated radon daughter levels and higher temperatures–the kind of place where (for example) white foremen stationed black workers in South African mines. The scientific (and apparently presentist and delocalized) question of causality–does radon cause cancer?" – is thus also, always, a historical and geographical question. It has no single, abstract answer above and beyond the politics of expert controversy, labor organization, capitalist production, or colonial difference and history.

References

Gabrielle Hecht, "Hopes for the Radiated Body: Uranium Miners and Transnational Technopolitics in Namibia," *Journal of African History* 51:2 (June 2010): 213-234.

Gabrielle Hecht, "Africa and the Nuclear World: Labor, Occupational Health, and the Transnational Production of Uranium," *Comparative Studies in Society and History*, 51/4 (October 2009): 896-926.

Funding support:

National Science Foundation Grant, Award # SES-0848568 , PI (2009-10).

National Endowment for the Humanities Fellowship (2009-10).

National Endowment for the Humanities Collaborative Research Grant, PI, with consultant Bruce Struminger (2004-07).

National Science Foundation Grant, Award # SES-0237661, PI (2003-04).

National Endowment for the Humanities Fellowship (2003-04).

Notions of Nature and the Debate over Vaccination in Late 20th Century US

Elena Conis
University of California, San Francisco, San Francisco, CA, USA

From the late 1970s through the 1980s, a growing number of American parents began to vocalize concerns about vaccines. The modern so-called anti-vaccine movement, still extant today, first coalesced around the revelation, in 1982, that pertussis vaccine carried a high risk of severe neurological side effects. But in the years before that scare, parents, some doctors, and other observers had already begun questioning the safety and necessity of vaccines generally. Among a host of other factors, their vaccine worries reflected a set of beliefs about the natural world and a set of ethics informed by the environmental discourse of their time.

Several historians have described the overlap between anti-vaccinationism and the concurrent vegetarian, food reform, and nature based health movements, such as the homeopathic movement, in the 19th century and early 20th century.[1] In the late 20th century, vaccine resistors were not just vegetarians and homeopaths, but their vaccine concerns did reflect the influence of a particular way of thinking about nature. This paper discusses four ways in which vaccine-critical rhetoric in the 1970s and 1980s was influenced by contemporary notions of nature and the environment. First, many who questioned vaccines at the end of the century worried that the trappings of modern life were toxic and disease promoting. Second, they categorized vaccines as modern technologies with unknown – but likely devastating – consequences for human health, and they were particularly concerned about the relationship between vaccination and the rising prevalence of chronic disease. Finally, these same critics often espoused an ecological view of health, were troubled by what they saw as the artificial nature of vaccination, and were concerned that vaccination represented a dangerous sort of tampering with otherwise benign nature.

These critiques of vaccination were linked to a larger set of sociopolitical critiques inspired by the social movements – including the feminist and consumer movements – of the 1970s. They also reflected a traditionally American discomfort with the expansion of state activities impinging upon personal lives and liberty. US vaccination efforts had grown significantly in the 1970s. Prior to then, a minority of states actively required children to be vaccinated against one or two infections to enroll in school. This gradually changed following the postwar development of new vaccines; a series of studies indicating the epidemic-thwarting abilities of school vaccine laws; and the implementation of federal vaccination-promoting policies. By 1981, every state had enforceable laws requiring students to be vaccinated against as many as seven infections.

This expansion was met with gradually mounting resistance, signaled by the 1974 republication of *The Poisoned Needle*, naturopath Eleanor McBean's 1957 diatribe against the smallpox and polio vaccines.[2] But the most visible forum for vaccine skeptics to emerge in the 1970s was Mothering, a new magazine catering to the back-to-the land sensibility of the new environmentalists. In the late 1970s, Mothering began to publish a range of dissenting voices on the issue of vaccination; in the 1980s, it became a key forum for the airing of vaccine critiques.

On the pages of Mothering, McBean lumped vaccines in with modern "poisons" – including "poison preservatives in foods and poison spray on farm produce." Mothering's readers expressed even greater concern about the chemical – as opposed to biological – components of vaccines. In letters to the magazine, they routinely referred to vaccines not as "poisons," but as "toxic," employing a term that had by then come into widespread use to describe the state of the modern environment. They drew parallels between vaccines and environmental chemicals, notably water pollutants and air pollutants, in addition to food preservatives, infant formula, and drugs administered during lactation and pregnancy. One critic, in a self-published pamphlet, provided readers with a list of toxic chemicals in vaccines, including the carcinogen formaldehyde and the mercury derivative thimerosal. "When cancer causing elements are found in foods, they are either banned (remember cyclamates?) or an obvious warning label appears on the package (saccharin, cigarettes)," she wrote. "There seems to be a double standard for vaccines."[3]

The influence of environmental discourse is clear on the pages of Mothering and anti-vaccine tracts published at this time. Vaccines were described as chemical time bombs, "witches' brews" of chemicals with uncertain "long-term consequences" which were tilting bodies and nature "out of balance." The term "artificial" was applied to vaccines with derision; critics saw natural encounters with infectious agents as a more well-defined and therefore preferable risk. Vaccines were thus linked to the host of postwar technologies that had proved harmful only after their widespread use; one critic thus called them "a sacrament of our...participation in the unrestricted growth of scientific and industrial technology."[4]

Vaccine skeptics also expressed the belief that vaccines were creating new diseases by taxing the immune system. They blamed vaccines for modern diseases with as-yet unexplained etiologies, including AIDS and escalating rates of allergies, lupus, and chronic fatigue syndrome. This fundamental idea evolved as it persisted through the turn of the century: vaccines were thought to cause cancer in the 1970s; SIDS, AIDS, and immune disorders in the 1980s; and in the 1990s, learning disabilities, ADD, asthma, multiple sclerosis, and autism. This preoccupation with unknown, long-term consequences of modern interventions links this history with episodes in the history of environmental health, including scientific and lay disputes over the effects of fluoride, radioactive fallout, lead, toxic waste, and DDT.

On the heels of the environmental movement, the parents and physicians who articulated vaccine skepticism in this period saw vaccination as an unwarranted meddling with nature, an artificial intrusion that resulted in weakened bodies out of balance with the natural order. They brought the chemical components of vaccines under harsh scrutiny, because these indicated that someday vaccines, like cigarettes, cyclamates, and saccharin before them, would be proven detrimental to long-term health. Their critiques embodied the widely held doubts of their day, namely, that the hubris of modern science and technology was unwarranted. As one critic put it in the pages of Mothering, vaccination amounted to an "attempt to beat nature at her own game, to eliminate a problem that cannot be eliminated...that is, the susceptibility to disease itself."[5]

References

[1] Durbach, Nadja. *Bodily Matters: The Anti-Vaccination Movement in England, 1853-1907*. Durham: Duke University Press; 2005.

[2] McBean, Eleanor. *The Poisoned Needle*. 3rd ed. Mokelumne Hill, CA: Health Research; 1974

[3] Cournoyer, Cynthia. *What About Immunizations?* Canby, OR: Concerned Parents for Information; 1983.

[4] Moskowitz, Richard. "Immunizations: The Other Side." *Mothering*, 1984: 32.

[5] *Ibid*, 37.

Musculoskeletal Disorders: A Long Way before Recognition, a Spectacular Course After: The French Case in the Twentieth Century

Nicolas Hatzfeld
University of Evry, Evry, France

Background

Periarticular pathologies offer a particular scope for examining different forms of historical aspects of occupational health, at the national and transnational levels. These diseases are linked to the movements made and to the postures adopted by workers, but it is sometimes difficult to individuate which part of these pathologies can be imputed to work. For this reason in particular, many States have for a long time avoided letting them feature on lists of illnesses for which compensation can be paid.

In the French case, a law authorizes in 1919 the compensation of recognized occupational diseases. However, the State Department of Labor does only in 1972 recognize one of the musculoskeletal disorders, and extends in 1982 and 1991 the right to compensation to various pathologies. During this long intermediate period, workers take action to obtain the compensation of their professional illness, in vain. Since the 1930s, the section in charge of the recognition asks itself about theses musculoskeletal overuse syndromes. After 1945, the officials of the French public welfare system frequently intervene in behalf of the recognition. But the Department of Labor, the medical experts and the officials of civil service refuse the recognition, using several arguments and administrative procedures. The building of European community at the beginning of the 1960s and the critical movement of the "1968 years" open the barrier of administrative denial.

During the 1980s and 1990s, alike the majority of industrial countries, France sees a spectacular rise in the incidence of periarticular work-related illnesses. This phenomenon shakes up the experts, the social groups and the political powers. Some trade unionists and researchers attempt to understand the phenomenon on an international scale. In France, they contribute to a public sensibility and to a relative evolution of the public policy in this field.

Materials and methods

Most of materials come from public archives: National archives of the French Departments of Labor and of Social affairs (1920-2000). Archives of the French public welfare system, of the European community (1957-1970), of National agencies for safety and health at work and for working conditions. The main reviews of health at work have been studied. For the last period, private archives have been used, mainly given by occupational health physicians and by experts of public agencies.

Conclusions

In the 19th century periarticular disorders were generally thought to be the inevitable concomitants of certain occupations or working-class modes of life. Yet surgeons in different countries, as well as a few physicians, came to be interested in the relationship between certain pathologies and the nature of activity, especially with regard to new occupations (typists, sewing-machinists, telegraphers...), and thus succeeded in establishing the role of work in the aetiology of certain types of disease.

The system of compensation for occupational disease eventually adopted in France in the early 20th century was however for a long time inimical to the victims of periarticular disorders, due to the Ministry of Labour's refusal to categorize these pathologies as compensable, while the ongoing negotiation between unions and employers' organisations in connection with the system was of no assistance, as a result of scientific uncertainty, employer resistance and the priority accorded by unions to other, more serious, diseases.

This refusal of recognition was also facilitated by the disaggregation of these diseases into specific types, in accordance with location, cause and affected occupation, and by the legal distinction between disease and accident, which excluded lesion due to repeated microtrauma.

The process of gradual recognition at first saw these isolating categories maintained intact. In the mid-1980s, however, the international dissemination of research led to growing recognition of the role of crosscutting factors, especially repetition, overexertion, and time constraint, a generalisation reflected in the emergence of the concept of "musculoskeletal disorders." This transnational dimension had two levels: on the one hand, international organisations such as the International Labour Office or the European Economic Community sometimes played a proactive role, while on the other, international awareness on the part of academics and experts accelerated the development of legitimately attested understandings.

Changes in understanding between 1985 and 2005 paralleled a change in the conditions of production of knowledge, now increasingly based on co-operation between workplace agents (occupational physicians, trade unionists, etc.) and official experts (ergonomists, epidemiologists, physiologists), the observations of the former prompting studies by the latter, generating results capable of modifying the categories of occupational disease established by the Ministry of Labour. Furthermore, the specialists overcame disciplinary differences to cooperate in joint investigations.

The observed proliferation of claims turned out to reflect only a fraction of the real incidence of periarticular disorders, studies regularly showing that there were far fewer claims than actual cases. Claims were however sensitive to changes of administrative definition, an observation that suggests prudence in interpreting the sometimes-spectacular differences in figures between countries and between different times in the same country.

In the French case, a very rapid growth in the number of cases over three decades corresponds to changes in work. More intensive, demanding and constraining models of work organisation are becoming more common. At the same time, the job market is getting tighter, bringing the growth of unemployment, the spread of precarious employment, and a reduction in the possibilities of occupational mobility. In this sense, the increase in musculoskeletal disorders may be said to reflect an accentuation of tensions in employment.

In general, then, the musculoskeletal disorders may be said to offer excellent evidence of how the boundary between the normal and the unacceptable in work-related disorders is socially defined.

The Ups and Downs of US Ergonomics Standards

David Rempel
Division of Occupational and Environmental Medicine
University of California, San Francisco, San Francisco, CA, USA

Musculoskeletal disorders account for the majority of disabling injuries in US workplaces. Yet there are no federal public health standards to prevent these injuries. In 2001, a scientific panel assembled by the National Academy of Sciences and the Institute of Medicine concluded that there was adequate evidence to support public health measures, using ergonomic principles, to prevent these disorders (NRC 2001). But a national ergonomics standard has failed to emerge.

The history of workplace ergonomics standards at the local and national levels is a complex one. Responding to pressure from unions, San Francisco, CA and Albany, NY introduced ergonomic regulations for computer users in the mid-1980s. This initial success encouraged unions to push for ergonomic regulations covering all industrial sectors. In the late 1980s, during the Reagan administration, OSHA issued multi-million dollar fines to the Big Three auto manufacturers for underreporting musculoskeletal disorders. These fines led to negotiated settlements between OSHA, the union, and the auto manufacturers that established robust ergonomic programs including management support, trainings, workplace changes, and assignments of responsibilities. Assembly lines were modified to reduce forceful hand and arm loading; these changes led to reductions in lost-time injuries.

This encouraged unions to petition federal OSHA for a national ergonomics standard. Rule making began in 1995. An ergonomics rule was published on November 13, 2000 during the last months of the Clinton administration (Federal OSHA, 2000). After intense lobbying from industry groups, the standard was repealed on March 7, 2001, one of the first acts of Bush II. Industry organizations were concerned that the standard was far reaching without clear criteria for enforcement.

During the same time period, in the 1990s, several states began the process of setting standards for ergonomics. In 1999, California became the only state in the country with an industry wide ergonomics standard (California Code of Regulations 1997). Washington State developed an ergonomics rule but it was repealed by a ballot referendum in 2003. Recently, some states have passed targeted ergonomics rules on safe patient handling in hospitals and nursing homes.

In parallel to these federal and state activities, consensus based, non-enforceable national ergonomics standards were developed separately by ANSI/HFES (American National Standards Institute/ Human Factors and Ergonomics Society; Z365 Committee) and the ACGIH (American Conference of Governmental Industrial Hygienists). The 13-year effort by ANSI/HFES was abandoned in 2001 following legal challenges from industry. The ACGIH established ergonomics guidelines (e.g., TLVs) for hand activity and lifting in 2001 after settling legal challenges from industry (ACGIH 2011). Many companies have voluntarily added ergonomics programs to their health and safety policies and have benefitted with reductions in lost-time injuries and workers' compensation costs and improved morale (GAO 1997).

Considering the method of the repeal of the 2000 rule and intense opposition from industry, it is unlikely that an industry wide federal ergonomics rule will be promulgated in the US. Instead, new ergonomics standards are likely to be developed by professional organizations, such as the ACGIH, or by states.

REFERENCES

American Conference of Governmental Hygienists. Threshold Limit Values and Biological Exposure Indices. ACGIH, Cincinnati, Ohio, 2011

California Code of Regulations, Title 8, Section 5110. Repetitive Motion Injuries. 1997.

Federal OSHA, Ergonomics Program; proposed rule. 29CFR Part 1910, Federal Register. March 7, 2000; 65 (45): 11948.

General Accounting Office. Worker Protection: Private Sector Ergonomics Programs Yield Positive Results. GAO/HEHS-97-163, General Accounting Office, Washington, DC, 1997.

National Research Council and Institute of Medicine. Musculoskeletal Disorders and the Workplace. National Academy Press, Washington, D.C., 2001.

Work-Related Neurobehavioral Toxicity from a Historical Perspective.

Roberto G Lucchini[1], Renato Gilioli[2]

[1] *Occupational Health, University of Brescia, Brescia, Italy*

[2] *Clinica del Lavoro, University of Milan, Milan, Italy*

"In Venice, on an island called Murano where large mirrors are manufactured, workers who use mercury show motor impairment . . . and with grim expression contemplate their sorrowful state in their mirrors . . . and detest the work that they have chosen." This was how Bernadino Ramazzini depicted in 1713 the effects of mercury, not only on motor function but also on mood. This might be an early start of the concept that exposure to toxic agents can cause effects on both neurological functions and behavior. In XIX century, experimental psychologists described human behavior by analyzing sensitivity to visual, auditory and other sensory stimulation. Sir Francis Galton (England 1822–1911) founded psychometrics and Emil Kraepelin (Germany 1856–1926) measured the psychological effects caused by the "external environment." The first description of neuro-behavioral toxicity such as "mercurial erethism" (Bateman et al.,1818) and "locura manganica" (Couper, 1837) date back to the same period, which is coincident to the development of industrial revolution.

Experimental psychology lead to neuro-psychology, that can be considered the other precursor of modern neurobehavioral toxicology. In the experiments of John B. Watson in 1914, Ivan Pavlov in 1927, Edward Thorndike in 1932, the brain was considered as organized in defined areas where association took place for the development of behavior, with no control by mental functions.

The dual dimension of "mind" and "brain" was revaluated and neuropsychology evolved from a "behaviorist" to a "cognitivist" discipline. The neuropsychological assessment entailed administration of stimuli and the assessment of performance in specific tasks, by measuring both the accuracy of responses (ratio correct/incorrect responses) and the reaction times. Specific tests developed and validated by traditional neuro-psychologists in cases of cerebral damage, were applied to clinically defined intoxications that were identified as "toxic encephalopathy." In 1930s a survey on the effects from exposure to carbon disulfide (CS2) was conducted in Pennsylvania with neuro-psychiatric interview on workers and their families. From 1960-1970 several psychological assessment were conducted in the Finnish viscose rayon plant by Helena Hänninen, and in similar plants in Germany and Italy (Cassitto et al., 1978). It was the official birth of "behavioral toxicology," although Hänninen preferred the term "toxico-psychology" since "it emphasizes psychology as the mother discipline" (Hänninen, 1985). Since 1970, the Psycho-physiology Research Unit in Sweden started the development of automated psychometric methods (Gamberale and Svensson, 1974). In the early seventies, unlike many areas of occupational health and occupational medicine which had already produced substantial information on methodologies to prevent and detect workplace disorders from chemical, physical and biological agents, the field of behavioral neurotoxicology was largely unknown. Along with changes in work technologies and working environment that reduced manual work while increasing mental and psychological effort, it was recognized that higher engagement of the nervous system activities deserved more information on possible adverse effect form exposure to neurotoxicants. Further, it became gradually possible to detect early changes in the brain that were indicated as "psycho-organic syndrome."

The first international meeting on Behavioral Toxicology was held at NIOSH in Cincinnati in 1973 by Charles Xintaras, Barry Johnson and Ido de Groot. That meeting indicated the need for a subsequent periodical review of the state of the art in this new discipline. It pointed out also the necessity of a common approach to neurotoxic effects in the work environment. Based on these premises, the newly restructured ICOH Scientific Committee on Neurotoxicology and Psychophysiology, in collaboration with the World Health Organization Headquarters in Geneva, sponsored a series of triennial symposia on neurobehavioral methods in occupational and environmental health. The first three symposia (Milan, 1982; Copenhagen, 1985; Washington DC, 1988) were aimed to exchange state of the art information on the development and application of neurobehavioral methods in occupational and environmental health by sharing experiences with colleagues from the developing countries, in order to devise preventive and medical strategies compatible with the resources. Regarding this issue, the previous symposia were mainly concerned with emerging problems in Africa and Latin America by trying to develop simple and inexpensive protocols and tools. Instead, the symposia which followed (Tokyo, 1991; Cairo, 1994, Shanghai, 1997) focused more on the respective Regions and addressed, with more emphasis, the issue of the effects on the nervous system functions. During these three symposia, specific topics included neurotoxic effects of industrial chemicals, use of neurobehavioral test batteries (WHO Neurobehavioral Core test battery) with special reference to cross cultural applications, recent electrophysiological neuroimaging techniques, biochemical markers, questionnaire studies, epidemiological studies of neurotoxic disorders, work-related stress and psychosomatic illness, current advances of the effects on the nervous system due to occupational and environmental factors. Later on, environmental and occupational factors versus aging and neurogenegerative illness in the elderly, educational strategies for prevention of work-related or environmental neurobehavioral effects became prominent themes. This new approach was reflected in the following symposia held in 1999 in Stockholm, Sweden, in 2002 in Brescia, Italy, in 2005 in Gyeongu, Korea, and in 2008 in San Josè, Costarica. All these initiatives contributed largely to disseminate information not only in industrialized countries where often a decrease of neurotoxic syndromes was observed, but also in underprivileged areas of the world, although these problems are far from being resolved and are still prevalent.

References

Bateman T. Notes of a case of Mercurial Erethism. *Med Chir Trans.* 1818; 9(1): 220–233

Cassitto MG, Bertazzi PA, Bulgheroni C. Subjective and objective behavioral alteration in carbon disupphide workers. *Med Lavoro.* 1978; 69:144-150

Couper J. On the effects of black oxide of manganese when inhaled into the lungs. *Br Ann Med Pharmacol.* 1837; 1: 41–2

Gamberale F, Svensson G. The effect of anesthetic gases on the psychomotor and perceptual functions of anesthetic nurses. *Work Environ Health.* 1974;11(2):108-13.

Hänninen, Twenty-Five years of Behavioral toxicology within Occupational Medicine: A personal account. *Am J Ind Med* 1985; 7: 19-30

Harriet Hardy and the Workers of Los Alamos

Ken Silver

Associate Professor of Environmental Health, College of Public Health, East Tennessee State University, Johnson City, TN, USA

Introduction

Dr. Harriet Hardy spent 1948 in the Occupational Health Group at Los Alamos Scientific Laboratory and continued to consult for the Atomic Energy Commission during her later academic career. Although her mentor and collaborator Alice Hamilton[1] has been the focus of extensive biographical research, Harriet Hardy has attracted little scholarly attention. Often credited with discovering beryllium disease in the Americas,[2] she became the first woman granted tenure at Harvard Medical School and had longstanding affiliations with Massachusetts state government and the Massachusetts Institute of Technology. She died in 1993 at the age of 88.

Methods

The contemporary campaign for the Energy Employees Occupational Illness Compensation Program Act (EEOICPAct) brought to the fore living Los Alamos retirees in whose cases of occupational illness Dr. Hardy played a pivotal role in diagnosis or case management. Official meetings in New Mexico in 1999 and 2000 between Los Alamos families and the U.S. Department of Energy (DOE) yielded cases of chronic beryllium disease and mercury poisoning. Methods of participatory action research were used to assemble and review extensive medicolegal documentation, with the aim of strengthening the workers' claims for compensation. These included: referral to occupational specialists intrigued by Hardy's involvement; collaboration with congressional district offices in making requests for medical records; and living room meetings to strategize in light of the evidence. Concurrently, a documents discovery project sponsored by the Centers for Disease Control, focusing on past environmental releases from Los Alamos, fostered an approach for stakeholder involvement which I call "Public History and

Public Health." A grassroots scientific poster session was held in Espanola, New Mexico in April 2003. In addition, fruitful searches were conducted of DOE's online Opennet database and Hardy's papers archived at Radcliffe's Schlesinger Library.[3] An additional case of beryllium disease, presumed deceased, was documented in an archive at the University of Tennessee.

Findings

These three cases would have remained shrouded by the DOE's "culture of secrecy" were it not for the field hearings on the proposed EEOICPAct initiated by the agency in 1999. Tellingly, it was not until a fourth request for records, in follow up to a congressman's tour of Los Alamos records facilities in 2006, that a microfilm image of Hardy's hand-written clinic intake notes from February 1948 was provided to the mercury poisoning claimant. Nor were Hardy's memos to superiors about dangerous mercury exposures included in the patient record; these were discovered on Opennet. And while several documents confirm the worker's recollection that a urinalysis for mercury was ordered by Hardy, the results thereof are curiously omitted from records provided to date.

The medicolegal histories of these cases, along with Hardy's diary entries, highlight opportunities and barriers in the early career of this leader in worker-oriented occupational health. Hardy integrated her cutting edge knowledge of clinical toxicology with her family upbringing steeped in debate and argumentation. These traits allowed her to provide leadership, both as an insider and an outsider, for institutions dominated by values of secrecy, denial and experimental physical science.

Prior to Hardy's arrival, the mercury case had visited the infirmary four times only to be told by another physician that he was "allergic" to something, then sent back to work. Hardy promptly visited the work area and four days later sent a memo to a supervisor recommending the mercury operation be shut down immediately and the work area cleaned. This generated "[l]oud complaints from those using mercury" in experimental work around Los Alamos.[4] The dispute reached Lab Director Norris Bradbury, who sided with Hardy in shutting down the operation.

As a Yankee woman at Los Alamos, she was an outsider, not yet part of the atomic culture of secrecy. According to her autobiography, Hardy argued at length with Los Alamos classification personnel over excessive secrecy. As a further sign of her alienation, near the end of her year at Los Alamos in November 1948 she wrote in her diary:

"I do not feel congenial with the disciplines of physics [and] mathematics...[T]here is a kind of inelasticity and narrowness to the minds of these men—more from training than the content of their fields; imagination is not part of their equipment... the admission of variables is not allowed..."

On February 22, in between visiting the mercury work area and recommending its shut down, she admits to her diary to being "homesick." Three weeks later she was "enjoying" social interactions with Louis and Eleanor Hempelmann, but with "reservations I can't define." Hempelmann was the physician leader of Health Division who had recruited her to Los Alamos. Perhaps her unease came from something which was not public knowledge until decades later: as early as 1945 he was one of the principal practitioners of secretive experimentation with plutonium on human subjects.[5]

Each contemporary conversation with the mercury case has been punctuated by the statement:

"She saved my life. I really believe that. If Dr. Hardy hadn't done what she done, I don't think I'd be alive today. The Lab wouldn't have done a thing."

After the 1948 episode, the mercury case worked 33 years in other areas at Los Alamos. So, his perception of Dr. Hardy's exceptionalism was likely influenced by interactions with later health and safety professionals.

Hardy's last New Mexico diary entry on Thanksgiving Day 1948 had a poignant tone: "As I depart I have had a very touchingly large number of apparently genuine and spontaneous expressions of compliment 'For what you have done,' and regret at my leaving, amounting to an accusation of desertion." She felt that workers' feelings of desertion originated in a "lack of leadership of my predecessors," specifically: "a lack of warmth of physician-worker/patient relationship that stems from the statistically-textbook-experimental:test tube kind of approach that has left my admissions feeling deserted..."

Decades would elapse – with many hazardous exposures incurred – before worker-centered advocates, informed by science, would effectively address the health concerns of Los Alamos workers in a climate of openness at the end of the twentieth century, quite different from the one challenged by Harriet Hardy in 1948.

References

[1] Hamilton, A. and Hardy, H.L. *Industrial toxicology*, 2nd ed. New York: P.B. Hoeber, 1949

[2] Zwerling, C., Salem Sarcoid: the origins of beryllium disease. In: Markowitz, G.E. and Rosner, D.. editors. *Dying for work: workers' safety and health in twentieth-century America*. Bloomington: Indiana University Press; 1987, pp. 103-116
[3] Harriet Louise Hardy Papers, MC-387. Schlesinger Library, Radcliffe Institute for Advanced Study, Cambridge, MA
[4] Hardy, H.L. *Challenging man made disease: the memoirs of Harriet L. Hardy, MD*. New York: Praeger, 1983
[5] Welsome, E., *The plutonium files: America's secret medical experiments in the Cold War*. New York: Dial Press, 1999

The "Invisible" Role of the Women's Movement for the Improvement of Working Conditions at the End of the Nineteenth Century: The case of Ersilia Majno Bronzini

Salerno Silvana
ENEA, Italian National Agency for New Technologies, Energy and Sustainable Economic Development, Rome, Italy

Introduction

The Italian women movement in the late of the nineteenth century was represented by Maria Montessori (1870-1952), Anna Kuliscioff (1853-1925), Alessandrina Ravizza (1846-1915), Sibilla Aleramo (1876-1960), Nina Sullam Rignano (1871-1945) and Ersilia Majno Bronzini (1859-1933) among many others. The women's occupational health, child labour and girls forced to "prostitution," were the mainstreams in the italian progressive women movement. In the Birmingham Conference on History in Occupational Health we discussed how Maria Montessori played an important role as a forerunner in ergonomics and occupational health. In this paper we focus the network of Ersilia Majno Bronzini (Majno Bronzini) towards the improvement of the workers'condition particularly women and minors.[1]

Methods

Most references were collected from the archives of the journal "Il Lavoro" (1901-1924), the archives of the association "Union of Women," its periodical (1901-1905) founded by Majno Bronzini and other material.

RESULTS

We found the Majno Bronzini's selected published papers on the working conditions of women and child labour claiming a national occupational health law. In the year 1880 Lombardy presented a picture of more women working than men (78,743 vs 24,438). Silk, cotton, linen and canvas industries employed many women and children less paid for the same job. In 1895 Majno Bronzini was asked to present a "Report on the work of women" at the Trade Union Congress in Milan;[2] in 1900 she expanded the previous paper for the Congress of Mutual Aid Societies in Milan and in 1902 she published "Towards a Law on the Work of Women and Child Labour" booklet containing all data on women unhealthy working conditions. Majno Bronzini dedicated herself particularly to improve the working conditions of girls called "piscinine" (meaning "very small" in the dialect of Milan). The "piscinine" of tailor and fashion shops received a pay of 20 to 50 cents for 11 to 14 hours of work per day. On June 1902, 250 girls organized a strike. They asked for a minimum wage of 50 cents, wage for hours working overtime, a limit of ten hours per day, weight regulation for the packages they had to handle. The "Unione Femminile" (Union of Women (UF)), founded in Milan on December, 1899, thanks to the efforts of Majno Bronzini, Nina Rignano Sullam and other women, supported the "piscinine" strike and they became supporters of the Association.

The education for women, the care of motherhood, infancy, work and legal self help were the UF main issues against the marital rule established by law. In 1902 the UF became a National Association with new branches throughout Italy. Among these the Roman branch was started by Sibilla Aleramo and Anna Frantzel Celli, wife of Angelo Celli (hygienist, malariologist, anthropologist). Anna Frantzel Celli and Majno Bronzini will share the same engagement as testified in the correspondence till 1925. The main UF activity in Rome was for the promotion of schooling and the struggle against malaria in the Roman Campagna and the Pontino Marshes, two sides of the same problem, and Maria Montessori's method was applied in those schools with her support. Later on, Maria Montessori corresponded to Majno Bronzini saying, "I have received the journal of the Union of women .... Please take me into account as a subscriber of the journal that is very interesting in all its parts, edited with simple and up to date issues."

In 1902 Angelo Celli officially congratulated Majno Bronzini's (and Anne Kuliscioff's) efforts to promulgate the first law on women and child labour during his speech before the Italian Parliament published by "Il Lavoro."[3]

Majno Bronzini network is also well kept in the letters (1901-1921)[4] she received from Luigi Devoto (1864-1936) (unfortunately we miss the letters of Majno Bronzini except two) after she started to get in touch with him at the end of the 1901, five years before the birth of the new institution "Clinica del Lavoro" in Milan.

Majno Bronzini, Nina Sullam Rignano, Elisa Boschetti (1869-1955) were among the supporter and organizer of the First Congress on Occupational illnesses in Milan (9-14 June 1906) where they were the only delegates of the flourishing women movement. Majno Bronzini, among professors and senators, signed the first petition against night shifts for women "Night work is against physiology and this is the reason why all ages, women and men particularly if under 18 years old, should be excluded."[5] Many years later Luigi Devoto in his journal "Il Lavoro" wrote the Majno Bronzini obituary considering her as a woman "Outstanding in Occupational Health" and "She was among the friends of the idea which leads us to the creation of the "Clinica del lavoro" and of "Courses on occupational illnesses in the years 1902-1903 at the Union of Women."[6]

After the First World War, Majno Bronzini coherently continued her commitment for the emancipation of women, from the abuse of unhealthy working conditions, from prostitution, from war and, at the end, from fascism till her death on the 17th of February 1933. In 1938, the UF was forced to close.

Majno Bronzini was very much in the tradition of women like Alice Hamilton (1869-1970) and Florence Kelley (1859-1932) who worked hard for progressive legislation and better working conditions. To place Italy in this comparative international perspective should be the key for future studies as Barbara Sicherman kindly suggested after this reading.

References

Salerno Silvana. An outstanding female figure in the history of occupational health: Ersilia Majno Bronzini. *Med Lav* 2010; 101 6: 419-426

Majno Bronzini Ersilia. Relazione sul lavoro delle donne. Milano Tipografia Milanese, Via Gesù 23, pagg. 32, 1900. Archivio Unione Femminile, Milano

Celli Angelo "Il lavoro delle donne e dei fanciulli." Discorso del prof. Celli pronunciato alla Camera il giorno 18 marzo 1902. Il Lavoro 1 (10) 153-159, 1901

Majno Edoardo "La Fondazione della Clinica del lavoro di Milano attraverso il carteggio Luigi Devoto-Ersilia Majno Bronzini" – Asilo Mariuccia – Centro di Ricerca e Documentazione per gli studi storici e sociali. Via Moisé Loira 77 -20144 Milano, 1985

Carnevale F., Baldasseroni A., Guastella V., Tomassini L. Concerning the First International Congress on Work related Illnesses-Milan 9-14 June 1906: success-news-reports-motions. *Med Lav* 2006; 97,2:100-113

Devoto L. (ascribed to) Una benemerita della Medicina del lavoro: Ersilia Majno Bronzini. Il Lavoro 2 (2) 79-80, 1933

Magic Bullet or Snake Oil? Aluminium Dust and the Prevention of Silicosis in Western Australia, 1938-1963

Criena Fitzgerald
Honorary Fellow, School of Humanities
University of Western Australia, Perth, Australia

This paper examined how aluminium dust was introduced into Western Australian Mines, the response of workers and the attempts by physicians to "enlighten" the Mines Department and the Industry about its true efficacy.

In March 1948, the Western Australian government amended the Mining Act to legislate that aluminium dust from the Canadian McIntyre Foundation be dispersed to underground gold mine workers to prevent silicosis. Although all mining companies understood that the suppression of quartz dust and good ventilation underground prevented silicosis, the Industry naturally favoured a "magic bullet," which would reduce the costs of mining and improve the productivity of the workforce and thereby increase profits. Aluminium therapy was one such "magic bullet," or quick fix that would, they hoped, reduce not only the production costs but also the costs of compensation for occupational disease in miners.

The McIntyre Foundation of Canada, which had investigated the treatment in animals in 1937, had already convinced the Canadian Government to make the inhalation of aluminium dust compulsory for Canadian miners. This was despite American evidence from Dr Leroy Gardner, an American authority on silicosis, "the prolonged use of Aluminium might produce harmful effects" on the lungs although there was no conclusive evidence. Confident of their own research findings, McIntyre Foundation representatives enthusiastically promoted the treatment for all miners and convinced the Western Australian Government to purchase its aluminium dust. In return the Western Australian Mines Department agreed to furnish silicosis statistics to the Foundation for its data and research.

The Mines Department, workers' compensation officials and the Australian Workers' Union (AWU) leaders were enthusiastic in their support of the new therapy, but rank and file miners were less keen to act as laboratory guinea pigs for an experimental treatment, which meant that they inhaled even more dust. Local mining inspectors reported that it was difficult for Inspectors to monitor the treatment because the "... discipline in the change rooms was very lax," and the attendant often released the powder and forgot all about it. At one inspection the Assistant Ventilation Inspector recorded the amount of time men stayed in the changerooms by recording their time on entry and exit and he found that most men frequently inhaled the dust for less than a minute. The response of a majority of the miners was eloquently described by ex machine miner Alan Walker, who recalled his shift boss stating:

> The Canadians invented this but there's been trouble with it. Nothing's been proven ... and ... as far as I'm concerned I've been on this mine for 30 years, I've sucked enough shit into my lungs without deliberately sucking somebody else's, some Canadians' bloody shit inside.

Despite such a disquieting and discouraging response, the Mines Department, the Chamber of Mines and particularly the AWU leadership persisted and continued to support the importation and use of aluminium dust.

This inconsistent state of affairs continued into the 1960s. Most miners continued to avoid exposing themselves to the dust for the required ten minutes; and many did not inhale the dust at all. In 1954, Mines Medical Officer Dr James McNulty concluded from an investigation of miners that the statistics showed that the prevalence and incidence rates of pulmonary tuberculosis, (including silico-tuberculosis) was much higher in goldminers than it should be in relation to other members of the community – despite the special supervision and preventative measures. He was openly critical of aluminium therapy. McNulty's report on the health of Western Australian miners articulated clearly the concerns of the medical profession, and in 1956, the Minister for Mines agreed to investigate the efficacy of aluminium therapy while on a forthcoming visit to America and Canada. He promised the Chamber of Mines that he would seek up to date statistics and information from "reliable sources outside the McIntyre Foundation." Despite this promise, nothing changed and the dust continued to be indiscriminately dispersed to an unknown number of miners.

For their part, public health doctors viewed the treatment as "snake oil," and about as effective, but until the establishment of the Occupational Health Division, they had no professional leverage over the Mines Department regarding silicosis prevention.

The Western Australian Division of Occupational Health in the Public Health Department had only been established in 1959 and it was under resourced and under funded. By 1961, however, its inaugural physician, Dr Letham began to assert his role as the State's occupational health physician. He wrote a position paper on Aluminium Therapy for the Public Health Department. After a brief literature review, he concluded that the experiments were poorly conceived and conducted, as were the therapeutic trials. He recommended the cessation of the therapy. It was only with a change in the leadership of the Australian Workers' Union (AWU) in 1963 that the treatment finally ceased.

No evaluation was ever undertaken. Aluminium therapy simply disappeared from Western Australian mines, the unused ejector in change rooms a lone reminder of the treatment. Unwilling to inhale yet more dust, miners passively resisted any attempts to make the treatment compulsory but all stated that they had inhaled the dust in order to avoid the possibility of losing compensation money. Their resistance, and the questionable statistics meant that the treatment could never be scientifically assessed, even if there had been medical support. Reluctant to endorse the treatment from the beginning, the Mines Medical Officer and later the Occupational Health physician became more vocal in their criticism. As early as the first year of operations, the Chamber of Mines began to have its doubts and efforts to encourage compliance remained unrewarded. Only the State Mining Engineer, and the AWU appeared to sustain their support for the treatment, and the AWU support only disappeared when the leadership changed in 1963. Aluminium therapy was no magic dust, or even magic bullet. Promoted by carpetbaggers or snake-oil salesmen, the best, as yet still unsubstantiated claim for the dust was that it appeared to do no harm!

The aluminium therapy programme undertaken by the Government of Western Australia was ill-conceived, politiclly and financially motivated, ineptly executed and never evaluated. It stands as an example of poor occupational health policy.

The research for this paper forms one chapter of Dr Fitzgerald's post-doctoral thesis 'Turning men into stone' Silicosis in Western Australia, as yet unpublished.

REFERENCES
Chamber of Mines Archive, various files, Item Nos. 6137, 6137A/156. JS Battye Library Western Australia.
State Records Office Western Australia, Mines Department Files.
State Records Office Western Australia Health Department Files.
Interview with Alan Walker 27/11/2008 by Criena Fitzgerald
Interview with Dr James McNulty 15/11/1992 by Criena Fitzgerald.
Aluminium Therapy File, Kalgoorlie Local Studies Collection, Kalgoorlie Western Australia.
Hogabom, Dieter Grant, 'Compensation and Control. Silicosis in the Ontario hard rock Mining Industry, 1921-1975', MA Thesis, Queens University Kingston, Ontario, Canada, 1997.

Miner's Asthma, Pneumoconiosis and the Politics of Occupational Disease in Coal Country, 1900-1970

Keirns CC.
Stony Brook University, Stony Brook, NY, USA

> At work you are covered with dust. It's in your hair, your clothes and your skin....You suck so much of it into your lungs that until you die you never stop spitting up coal....Slowly you notice that you are getting short of breath when you walk up a hill. On the job, you stop more often to catch your breath. Finally, just walking across the room at home is an effort.... Call it miners' asthma, silicosis, coal workers' pneumconiosis—they are all dust diseases with the same symptoms.
> *Lorin Kerr, Director of Occupational Health for the United Mine Workers of America, speech to UMW convention in 1968*[1]

Occupational lung diseases are now synonymous with both textile manufacture and mining, but a century ago there was an odd silence across coal country. From the 1880s through the 1940s, the Kentucky and West Virginia medical Journals published 4 articles on 'asthma' between them, and none on occupational lung diseases, miners' asthma, or pneumoconiosis. This silence is particularly stark in light of the fact that in the same period both states reported "asthma" mortality rates several times the national average, nearly 10-fold higher for men, and more than 25-fold higher for men listed as "colored" in Kentucky.

Despite the prevalence of respiratory disease in coal country, opinions abounded such as this one from the Cabell County, West Virginia Medical Society: "...a consensus of medical authority considers simple, uncomplicated, and uninfected coal workers' pneumoconiosis a condition compatible with reasonable health and not associated with significant disabling disease."[2] These views were challenged by physicians who worked for organized labor. In 1968, Donald Rasmussen, physician at the Appalachian Regional Hospital in Beckley, West Virginia (founded 1956 as part of the United Mine Workers', Miner's Memorial Hospital Association) reported that: "Physiologic studies of 192 symptomatic bituminous coal miners from one Southern Appalachian region... demonstrated significant pulmonary insufficiency in large numbers of subjects with only minimal roentgenographic evidence of pneumoconiosis."[3]

The country as a whole saw peak crude asthma mortality in 1951 at 4.63 per 100,000, nearly four times the rate seen in 2006. While asthma rates fell nationally from 1951-1978, bronchitis, emphysema and especially the new term chronic obstructive pulmonary disease began to be used in other regions in this period, and appeared to displace the term "asthma" somewhat in the mortality statistics. Overall respiratory mortality rose unabated to the range of 41 per 100,000 to 45 per 100,000, in the past decade.[4]

The story in coal country was quite different. Asthma rates remained persistently high among men in West Virginia and Kentucky until the late 1960s, while mortality attributed to pneumoconiosis was extremely rare as it was nationally, never more than 0.5 deaths per 100,000. After 1969 saw the passage of the Federal Coal Mine Health & Safety Act, the frequency of diagnoses reversed in the mortality statistics. From 1978 to the present, West Virginia and Kentucky have seen asthma mortality rates consistent with the national trends. Death certificates bearing the term pneumoconiosis, however, rose dramatically from less than 20 deaths per year to pneumoconiosis mortality of 6 to 7 per 100,000 (peaking in 2000 at 7.7 per 100,000 in West Virginia), higher than the highest recorded national asthma mortality rate, and more than 10 times the rates reported a generation ago, despite a substantial fall in the number of coal miners.

Many skeptical physicians, businesspeople, lawmakers, and bureaucrats have seen this rise in reported disease and attributed death in response to compensation as taking advantage of the federal compensation program. But an exploration of the practices of the period reveal a large burden of chronic respiratory disease, much of which was already being attributed to coal mining by both workers and their physicians, but under the older term "miner's asthma," that was now accounted "pneumoconiosis." The "structured silence" over occupational lung diseases in America's coal country in the first half of the twentieth century, was driven not just by employers resisting provision of compensation, but also by physicians who saw no reason to differentiate one lung disease from another. The available pharmaceuticals were and are shared across all of the chronic respiratory diseases, giving physicians little reason to distinguish them.

The story did not end with passage of the federal compensation program in 1969. Richard Nixon had been shamed into signing the Coal Mine Health & Safety Act by picketing widows from a mine disaster, and his Social Security Administration had no interest in implementing it. Criteria were quickly devised to process claims which required, besides documentation of occupational exposures which might have happened decades before, x-ray evidence of dust deposition in the lungs. Even a cursory examination of the history of silicosis shows that the difference between silica deposition and other dust diseases is the unusual visibility of silica dust on an x-ray, while coal dust, cotton dust, and many other organic and industrial dusts are only demonstrable at autopsy.[5] These criteria led to the denial of compensation to 60,000 miners in the first 3 years of the program. By 1972, coal miners and their advocates had returned to Congress seeking specific clarification of the criteria for compensable lung disease, clarification of Congressional intent that opened the compensation program to larger numbers of coal miners past and present, no matter what they had called their disease.[6]

References

[1] Lorin E. Kerr, Black lung. *Journal of Public Health Policy*, March 1980; 1(1): 50-63, quotation p. 50.

[2] Quoted in Sherrill RG. West Virginia Miracle: The Black Lung Rebellion. *The Nation*, 1969, 208: 529-30.

[3] Rasmussen DL, Laqeur WA, Futterman P, Warren HD, Nelson CW. Pulmonary impairment in southern West Virginia coal miners. *American Review of Respiratory Disease* 1968; 98: 665.

[4] Mortality, Washington, DC: US Bureau of the Census, series 1900-1936. Vital Statistics of the United States, Washington, DC: Government Printing Office, issued 1937-1993, subsequently online.

[5] Rosner D & Markowitz G. *Deadly dust: silicosis and the politics of occupational disease in twentieth-century America*. Princeton: Princeton Univer-

sity Press, 1991.
[6] Derickson A. *Black lung: anatomy of a public health disaster*. Ithaca: Cornell University Press, 1998.

Storming the Citadel: Popular Epidemiology and Scientific Innovation in British Silicosis Research

Joseph Melling
Centre for Medical History, University of Exeter, Exeter, UK

In 1937 Dr. A.J. Cronin published a novel about a young Scottish doctor working in south Wales mining towns who investigated lung disease among anthracite colliers before leaving to work as a research officer with the medical elite who controlled the "Coal and Metalliferous Mines Fatigue Board" in London. The Citadel drew directly on Cronin's own experiences as a young physician in south Wales and as medical inspector with the Mines Department as well as contemporary research on silicosis and pneumoconiosis. This novel appeared was published at a moment when medical understanding of miners' lung disease was about to be transformed with the appointment of a new research investigation by the independent Medical Research Council (MRC) into dust-related pulmonary illness among anthracite miners in south west Wales. Yet an international congress in 1930 had appeared to confirm the primacy of silica as a hazardous mineral and silicosis as the "king" of industrial diseases.

These changes took place in a setting of industrial, political and intellectual struggle during the late 1930s as trade union leaders, medical advocates and labour campaigners pressed for fresh investigation. The famous MRC survey of 1937-41 resulted in a radical reappraisal of what became known as coal workers' pneumoconiosis and greatly extended the scope of industrial compensation for dust-related disease in coal mining. Many historians have seen the overturning of the scientific orthodoxy as a testament to the success of a "lay epidemiology," based on the practical experience of workers, in the face of scientific denial, scepticism and collusion with industrial interests. The idea of "lay" or "popular" epidemiology has been recently applied to a wide range of historical case studies in a variety of industries and countries. These range from silicosis to asbestosis and they involve not only studies of workers but environmental activists and a range of political agents whose concern for the welfare of local communities enabled them to influence policy and the behaviour of powerful corporations.

This paper does not dispute the importance or the moral purpose of such activists but it raises questions about the way in which historians sometimes record, even celebrate, the achievements of such groups and portray the conservative inclinations of the scientific community at different periods. It is suggested here that scientific communities are as likely to be divided by political and moral questions as organisations of labourers or environmental activists. There is clearly no simple logic or analysis which arises from the wide diversity of everyday, or reflected, experience of different groups at different periods of history. Rather, knowledge is understood through cultural and ethical codes just as political initiatives arise from the combined choices of different groups. The emphasis here is on the formation of different networks of people, ranging from workers to scientists, insurers and employers, and their concern to understand the risks and hazard and their own likely liability to suffer from such hazards.

This perspective is developed in a fresh analysis of the British case in the period of the Medical Research Council's survey, commenting on technical as well as medical and industrial evidence, and offers a sceptical review of some arguments in regard to "lay epidemiology." It is suggested here that we need a careful analysis of divisions within the scientific and medical communities as well as labouring populations when we reconstruct the range of experiences, opinions and motivations of those groups most involved in the reappraisal of silicosis in the mid-twentieth century. Just as Cronin's novel is a moral fable based on personal experience so historians should register their own moral concerns and be sensitive to their subjective values in composing these hazardous histories.

Grindstone City's Second Product Silicosis, the Plausibility of Export of Dust Disease

Mary Lynn Zaremba, Alicia Redford, Kristin Elliott, Sridhar P. Reddy
St. Clair Pulmonary & Critical Care, P.C., Port Huron, MI, USA

Various sources of information are needed to ascertain the plausibility and to confirm disease including death records and medical information. When such data doesn't exist the "Old-Timer" becomes your only source. The number of people that were at risk for silicosis and those exposed or affected are not credibly known due to poor record keeping, poor understanding of the disease in the past and time from exposure to diagnosis. We looked at plausibility of the export of silicosis.

A Blind Hog's Acorns by Carey McCord MD book published in 1945, has an old- timer account of the rise and fall of Grindstone City and its relevance to silicosis. Grindstone City in Michigan, the United States of America had a reputation of the finest grindstones in the world and from 1835 to 1938 this grindstone was exported to far off places such as Japan and Germany. In 1938, production stopped due to the discovery and increasing use of silicon carbide as an abrasive material by Acheson in Ohio. Silica has been acknowledged as a cause of respiratory disease since ancient times. Hippocrates described lung disease in miners around 400 BC. While in 1713, Bernardo Ramazzini noted asthma type symptoms and sand-like substances in the lungs of stone cutters.

Mr. Joseph Summerville born in 1921 was our old-timer who lived in Grindstone City as a teenager. He was our main source along with pictures and other accounts. Grindstone City is located in the thumbnail tip of Michigan's mitten shaped contour.

In 1838, Captain Peer looking for goods for his ship came upon the perfect grindstone. On one trip, the sailors rigged up a crude fashion of stone slab and used it to sharpen their tools. That year (1838) Capt. Peer, getting the idea from the sailors began shaping the grindstones at this place now known as Grindstone City. The industry was carried on for nearly one century by Capt. Peer and several other people and companies.

Grindstones from Grindstone City were near perfect for their time, containing hard fine granules free from hardheads (embedded pebbles). They were exported to far off places such as: Russia, China, Japan, Canada, Africa and Germany. Up to 25,000 tons of grindstones a year was exported. Bolle's Industrial history of the United States supports some stones measuring 7 feet in diameter and 13 inches thick weighing about 2 tons. Huge stones from the Grindstone City measuring 7 feet in diameter were used up in 3 weeks to sharpen axe blades. It is plausible that this resulted in high silica exposure and probably caused silicosis.

Stones were mined and shaped by various processes including turning, trenching, drilling, reaming, blasting, wedging, and afterwards they were eyed, chipped and dressed. Gang saws, power chisels and steam powered rim cutters were utilized and turned on lathes being done by hand. Turning a stone means to carve the rock into a flat, round grindstone. To do this, the stone was first hauled to the mill where it would be finished. Here another steam engine was used to pick up the stone and it was guided by men to a machine called a mandrill, where it was put on a large iron bar and securely fastened there by bolts and washers. However, due to the hole in the stone, ropes instead of cables were used in this operation. Men stood on each side of this stone, which was upright on the bar. With long iron tools held against the stone, they cut the sides and edges of the stone. These tools were kept sharpened by the blacksmith who worked in a small building close to the mill. These tools looked similar to crowbars. The stone was kept turning by means of a steam engine and pulleys, and the men held their tools against the side of the stone as it turned, thus cutting and shaping it. When they had done one section they moved the tool forward to the next spike, until they had turned it to the center. The stone had to be exact for perfect balance or they would not be saleable.

The Americans considered fishing a good job at that time. Grindstone City died and became essentially a vacation / fishing village in 1936. The Lovejoy and Summerville families started a fishing business in Grindstone City in the 1920's. The French Canadians took the dustiest jobs of dressing and turning the stones in confined places also considered the worst jobs and had the highest paying jobs in town. They worked a few years and then went home to linger and die usually by age 40. Americans would not work in these rooms.

Except for old-timers accounts such as our old-timer Joseph and Carey McCord's MD old-timer "Old Angus McCachen" about silicosis in Grindstone City no other historical accounts exist that we are aware of. The ghost town of Grindstone City did seem to contribute to the burden of dust disease depicted by old-timers as grit consumption, dust on the lungs, rock tuberculosis, grinder's consumption or that weird disease that the doctors now call silicosis. Edward G. Acheson in 1891 while trying to make diamonds in a plumber's crucible made carborundum (silicon carbide) and mortally wounded Grindstone City. Ironically, the Acheson Family set up business in Port Huron, Michigan ninety miles away.

Grindstones from Grindstone City no longer contribute to burden of disease. Currently in Port Huron, Michigan grindstones adorn, as landscape rock, the local fast food restaurant. The near perfect grindstone of the past now highlights the next public health crisis "what is the icon in our Fast Food Nation" and its export around the world.

References

McCord CP. *A blind hog's acorns*. Chicago: Cloud Inc., 1945.

Italian Workers' Health Between the Two World Wars

Baldasseroni A,[1] Carnevale F,[1] Iavicoli S,[2] Petyx C,[2] Tomassini L.[3]
[1] *Local Health Unit of Florence, Florence, Italy.*
[2] *ISPESL, Italian National Institute for Occupational Safety and Prevention, Rome, Italy.*
[3] *University of Bologna, Bologna, Italy.*

Introduction

Italy, unified between 1860 and 1870 as a nation, suffered for old backwardness and chronic lacks. The illiteracy was the rule, not the exception at least in the greatest mass of the working population, the peasants. However at the end of the XIX century something was changing. The Italian ruling classes after the unification, had completed one clearly liberist choice that had carried to destroy important parts of the industrial apparatus as an example in the iron and steel field. However, the same liberals had quickly built up infrastructures, railroads and ports, modernizing in such way the economy and putting the country in connection with Europe. The 1906 International Milan exhibition was devoted to celebrate the conclusion of an extraordinary enterprise for the age, the Simplon tunnelling, more than 19 kilometres in length, wonder of railway engineering and pride of the Italian work.

The First World War interrupted such a development of Italian economy, and after the end of war turmoil and Squadrismo (Fascism rioting) erupted as a reaction to socialist uprising in factories of Northern Italy. Mussolini's movement begun with a sort of liberalism without rules destrying workers' movement. Then he built up the totalitarian State, imposing harmony between employers and employees through promulgation of "Carta del Lavoro" (Chart of Labour) and the development of "Corporativismo."

Discussion

Workers' health policy provides an important indicator to assess the whole range of social policies adopted during Fascism and to focus on the historical issue of continuity/discontinuity from Fascism to post-war democratic state, widely discussed at national and international level.

The safeguard of workers' health became pivotal as the Fascist regime, after an initial liberal phase, launched a series of social policies that soon turned into the ideological scheme and identifying mark of Fascism. With overwhelming propaganda Fascism accredits the hypothesis of work as an ethical value and the pivotal role of the worker. The Duce personifies this propaganda with a series of disguises that portray poses peasants and workers at their side.

During this period, public health and health at work had very different path. In the realm of public health, through the support of social insurance, social and hygienic improvements are guaranteed to the proletarian masses, instead of health and safety at work, where lack of intervention by the State went on the role of ruler and controller of working conditions is abandoned, and with the birth of ENPI (National Institute for Propaganda against Injuries), employers themselves are practically delegated to perform these tasks. The reformed and underfunded Corporate Inspectorate, follower of Labour Inspectorate, ensures the "harmonious" partnership between the parties.

One consequence is to emphasize the human factor in the genesis of industrial accidents, blaming the worker, not conscious of his role of "soldier of production."

Health protection became one of the official and institutional instruments to get "consensus."

The Fascist policy on workers' health protection was deeply inspired by the ideology and general policy of the Fascist corporative state and based on the collaboration between capital and labour and the creation of the "authoritative modernization"; in addition, the strict workers' health and safety issues brought to light at least two clear contradictions.

Case studies

There was lack of initiatives against exposure to toxic in workplaces. Medicalization and insurance against industrial diseases dominated. The context of production was characterized by backward and not original level of technology, reduction of wages and large amount of disposable workers. Production technological solutions were tested with no hygienic or medical control, if not after the incurrence of health damage. Even in these cases, tendency was to control the acute poisonings, allowing chronic development of diseases, complying with persistence of productive capacity. In some cases partial compensation insurance and welfare for the veterans of the work battles was allowed.

During the interwar period new epidemics emerged in Italy. Viscosa, artificial silk production picked since early twenties and Carbon disulphide intoxication was spread among female workers. The dyes industry, aromatic amines based, grew up in parallel with the increasing production of textiles and workers in this industry experienced the same well-known consequences of exposure to these chemicals as in Germany or Great Britain many years before. Benzene, bone-marrow toxicant, was used with no barrier to contact with workers mainly in medium and small factories and workshops. Silicosis crisis was evident in metallurgic industry at the end of the thirties, before any compensation right was established. Asbestos was largely mined with no specific hygienic regulation, i.e., general ventilation duty like in other countries (Great Britain in 1931). All this epidemics were well described into the scientific medical literature and in clinical case reports, mainly after the insurance coverage of a short list of industrial maladies. Very scarce was the contribution to knowledge of technical prevention by industrial hygiene.

Another clear contradiction lays in the gender issue and the so called "race defence," particularly relevant in the 30s. Long before Fascism turned into an overtly racist regime, health protection was pivotal in its family support strategies; in particular, women's health protection was strengthened because women, as mothers, safeguarded the pureness and the strength of the "Italic progeny." Nevertheless, the impetus towards eugenics and demographic growth collided with the awful working conditions and the inadequate protection measure for female workers. These issues led to a series of institutional changes which redefined the state interventions in this area; however, the regime's ability to actually implement such new tools proved to be quite limited.

Conclusions

Industrialization in Italy during Fascism is accomplished without taking any account of the experience of other countries that had preceded in the field of occupational health. The alleged primacy of "Italianity" (Ramazzini was wrongly cited) does not preserve the Italian workers from the deleterious effects of industrialization as well developed. In fact there is a continuity in the attitude of the State towards the protection of workers that can be found almost unchanged both before and after Fascism. The workers' movement fights at the end of the sixties broke down this trend.

References

Bianchi B, *I tessili: lavoro, salute, conflitti. In: Annali della Fondazione GG Feltrinelli, La classe operaia durante il fascismo*. Milano: Feltrinelli, 1981, pp. 973-1070.

Carnevale F, Baldasseroni A, *Mal da lavoro. Storia della salute dei lavoratori.* Roma-Bari: Laterza, 1999.
Gentile E, La *Grande Italia: The Myth of the Nation in the Twentieth Century.* Madison: University of Wisconsin Press, 2009.
Sapelli G, *Organizzazione del lavoro e innovazione industriale nell'Italia tra le due guerre.* Torino: Rosemberg & Sellier, 1978.
Willson PR, *The Clockwork Factory: Women and Work in Fascist Italy.* Oxford: Oxford University Press, 1993.

Occupational Health and Safety in Australia: The International Context 1900-1939

Rod Noble
School of Health Sciences, University of Newcastle, Newcastle, Australia

This paper is part of a larger work in progress that focuses on the institutions, organisations and practice of Occupational Health and Safety (OHS) in Australia from 1850s – 2000s. This larger work also outlines the international context within which Australian developments took place and identifies important links between them.

This expanded abstract concentrates on the period up to1939 and looks at the workplace relationships of the main stakeholders in relation to Occupational Health and Safety (OHS). It also looks at some OHS organisations that developed in the period; the similarities of developments occurring in other countries; forces within and without the workforce in relation to OHS, and the role of various professions.

Background

Occupational Health and Safety (OHS) has been the focus of activity in the workplace in Australia from at least the mid 1850s and in the 19th century this activity came primarily from within the workforce. It is fair to say that OHS was a significant element present at the very beginning of some sections of the organised labour movement in Australia.

Research has confirmed a gap between OHS corrective actions deriving from within the workplace and OHS actions directed at the workplace from outside. The first preceded the latter by many decades.

In Australia (and elsewhere in the world), in the 19th century, there was not a great deal of meaningful communication between the working class (including their organisations) and the employers. The latter dominated government and industry and it could be described as being like co-existing parallel worlds.

OHS activity from within the workplace

One of the most significant and earliest unions in Australia, the Miners Union, started because of an OHS issue.

In 1858, a mass meeting of miners from individual Lodges decided to campaign to improve ventilation in mines, they petitioned the Parliament for the appointment of an inspector of mines [Turner 1982]. There was a poor response from Government and employers to these campaigns. In 1860, the miners combined their Lodges into a Miners Association to have more leverage on these issues.

The miners in this period realised that ventilation was crucial both in the longer term, to lessen the risk of black lung, and the shorter term, to lessen the risk of explosions.

Workers were active from the beginning on the question of workplace health and safety preventative strategies, not just compensation. The campaign for adequate ventilation carried on for 50 years alongside the fight for workers compensation.

Miners even ran their own candidates for Parliament in the 19th Century, in part on safety issues. Rehabilitation and compensation was nonetheless also an important focus and many regional hospitals started out as miners hospitals, sustained by a union organised levy on miner's wages.

The workforce in the mining industry step up preventative action

Partly as a result of a terrible 1923 mining disaster in the Hunter Valley of New South Wales, the Miners Union, in 1924, moved to set up "Safety Propaganda Committees" on the coal fields for the purpose of directing public opinion towards unsatisfactory methods being used.

These committees arranged public lectures and distribution of literature on the question of safety in mines and pushed to set up a Royal Commission into Mine safety.

In January 1925 the Coal Mining Safety Propaganda Committees had a Conference in Newcastle, New South Wales where among other things they discussed the need for Mines Rescue Stations and the problem of "spontaneous combustion" in the thick seams of the local coal fields.

Workers and management in the steel industry: a parallel universe

In the 1930s management at an Australian steel works set up safety committees in the works. There was a central safety department that met each week, and, safety committees in each department presided over by a superintendent. Also, in the 1930s, it was reported in local press that the steel works management placed great importance on safety precautions. [NMH July 1939]

In the same period, a Trade Union Council report when noting accident rates in the same steelworks, referred to it as an "Abattoir." The report noted that up to 800 accidents requiring first aid were recorded at that steelworks in one particular week. The reasons recorded for this was a speed up in operation which in turn caused physical exhaustion and lack of vigilance. The report drew a direct link between the push for greater productivity, and a production bonus system, and the high rates of injury. [NTHC 1936]

The steelworks management on the other hand quoted unidentified safety "experts" who apparently contended that the human mind was constituted in such a way that only one idea could be the centre of attention at the one time. Management concluded that more than half the accidents at the same steelworks had been traced to this human limitation. [NMH1939]

One of Trade Union Council criticisms of the OHS Committees at the steelworks was that the committee was selected by the departmental superintendents. Thus they were a form of management control. Selected workers were called in to deliberate with their foreman and managers, and to lay complaints against them for not observing safety regulations. Of course none but the most courageous worker would do such a thing in view of the fear of dismissal. Subsequently, safety committees rarely functioned effectively. The Trade Union Council called for safety committees controlled by the workers to police safety regulations.

OHS activity from outside the workplace

There were OHS interventions of various kinds from outside the workplace, notably by the government through legislation. In the 1870s and 1880s, significant factory legislation was introduced into the various Australian colonies. Much of this legislation originated in Britain. There were also some management, medical, engineering and civil society/industry interventions.

In March 1916, in the Hunter Region of New South Wales a "Safety First

Movement" was established to begin work in the Railways and Tramways. The founder of this movement spoke of the need to prevent suffering brought about by lack of thought. He drew on experiences in the UK and USA. As an accident prevention method, the emphasis was on getting workers to alter their behaviour rather than make the workplace safe. This movement rarely sprung from the target workforce itself. It often consisted of people of position and influence in society who sometimes had quite altruistic reasons for their involvement.

In June 1926 a Mr J. K. MacDougall, addressed the issue of Industrial Safety from an employer's perspective at a meeting in the Hunter Valley. He was associated with the management of the local steel works. Many of his ideas came from the USA where he had recently visited and they were similar to that eventually pursued by the steelworks management itself in the 1930s as noted above.

Though there were some exceptions, medical doctors, architects and engineers tended to be reactive rather than proactive during this period. Factories and equipment were designed to be functional and to produce goods as required rather than optimise worker's health and safety. Again with exceptions, the medical profession tended to treat injuries and not pursue the cause. In a general sense, there was a social and physical separation of the working class, their organisations, and the professionals mentioned, and the latter were the people who were potentially able to play a greater role. This remained just a potential for a long time.

Conclusions regarding OHS activity from within the workplace

From the beginning the workers were not only interested in funeral benefits, hospitals and compensation. Evidence shows that workers and their organisations have had a long engagement with preventative strategies in regard to occupational injury and illness. Workers and management viewed the OHS situation in opposing ways.

Conclusions regarding OHS activity from outside the workplace

Outside intervention in the period being viewed tended towards safeguarding against failure of the human element, and to devise methods that would enable workers to safeguard themselves. Concepts of systematic OHS management as we would know them today were either not evident or in a very primary form. The emphasis of intervention from outside the workplace was strongly on modifying the worker, not the workplace.

General conclusions

The movement to improve Australian workplace safety started in the workplace in the 19th century from organised Workers and that aspect is still continuing. Engineering professionals became involved in various safety organisations – mostly from early 20th century.

Medical professionals became involved by first treating the results of workplace accidents and later by engagement with preventative measures.

Industrial management in Australia picked up safety ideas from various parts of the world and tried to apply these ideas in the Australian context. These ideas were a mixture of control strategies designed to maximise profits along with some prototype systematic OHSM, e.g., management commitment; procedures to monitor OHS conditions; control measures; evaluation.

References

Aldrich, Mark *History of Workplace Safety in the United States, 1880-1970*, Smith College.

Berman, D M *International Journal of Health Services* 1977; 7(1): 63-87.

Frick, K & Wren, J (2000), Reviewing OHS Management – multiple roots, diverse perspectives & ambiguous outcomes. Pp. 17- 42 in Frick, K. Jensen, L.P. Quinlan, M & Wilthagen, T (Eds) *Systematic OHS Management: Perspectives on an International Development*, Amsterdam, Pergamon Elsevier Science.

Newcastle Morning Herald, 6/3/1916, 9/6/1926, 8/7/1939.

Newcastle Trades Hall Council "Metal" Industry Report (1936).

Noble, Rod (2009), A History of OHS in Australia: a work in progress, unpublished.

Noble, Rod (2007), *A History of OHS in the Hunter Valley of NSW*, University of Newcastle.

Palmer, Lew (1926), History of the Safety Movement, *Annals of the American Academy of Political and Social Science*, Vol. 123, Jan 1926.

The History of the American Society of Safety Engineers 'Safety Through the Decades' . From: http://www.asse.org/about/history/php accessed 8-10-09.

Turner, John (1982), *Coal Mining in Newcastle 1801-1900*, Newcastle History Monograph No 9, Newcastle City Council.

Science and sales: Marketing the Pesticide DBCP in the Mid-20th Century United States

Susanna Rankin Bohme

Deputy Editor, International Journal of Occupational and Environmental Health, Attleboro, MA, USA

Introduction

As synthetic pesticide sales skyrocketed during the 1940s and 1950s, the new chemicals seemed to many to promise agricultural bounty and scientific control over nature. Utopian hopes for the new pest control were, however, countered by some scientists' and laypeople's concerns about the health and environmental effects of the chemicals. The chemical industry's major responses to these concerns were to integrate toxicological testing into the pesticide development process and provide consumers with warnings about the potential health risks of pesticides. As burgeoning science of toxicology was used to test the effect of new compounds on laboratory animals, it was also mobilized in industry public relations materials to assert that pesticides were subject to the careful controls of science before they could come in contact with the human body. The chemical industry also developed voluntary guidelines on warning practices, based on the idea that warnings could communicate the salient points of a chemical's dangers to a potential user. By allowing a rational individual to make an informed decision about whether and how handle the chemical, warnings helped shift the rhetorical—and some hoped, legal—responsibility for safety on to the user. New federal regulations on pesticide use and food residues were also based on the notion that citizens could be protected from the risks of pesticides through examination of unbiased, objective scientific data.

Toxicology and warnings seemed to resolve the contradictions between the promise of scientific control of pests and the frightening dangers posed by pesticides. However, the early history of the nematicide dibromochloropropane (DBCP) shows how the language and practice of science were mobilized to create a market for this pesticide both before testing was completed and after the emergence of disturbing toxicological evidence. When toxicological inquiries showed testicular damage and other problems in experimental animals, scientists worked together to downplay evidence of harm in order to secure regulatory approval and therefore avoid disruption of plans to sell the chemical.

Science In Dbcp Marketing

In the 1950s, DBCP was produced, tested and marketed by Shell Chemical Corporation and Dow Chemical Company. Contrary to industry claims that toxicological testing was conducted before pesticide compounds were marketed, Shell sold its "Nemagon" brand DBCP in 1955, and Dow followed with "Fumazone" two years later. Most farmers were not familiar with the wormlike soil-dwelling pests called nematodes that the chemical was meant to control, so marketing strategies included teaching farmers about the existence of the pests in order to convince them DBCP was not only necessary, but would increase farm earnings. The companies attempted this through a varied marketing campaign that mobilized the language of science and emphasized themes of control and abundance. Shell sponsored a series of "Nematology Workshops." Complete with a roster of academic and government experts, as well as corporate employees, the workshops were framed as technical seminars, but were used as platforms to promote DBCP and Shell's other nematicide product, DD. In its marketing, Dow used field demonstrations that took on the cache of scientific experimentation by producing tangible evidence of Fumazone's efficacy. Other marketing efforts used the language of science to reframe traditional farmer knowledge as inadequate to modern agriculture, which required expert diagnosis and chemical control. Advertising narratives linked scientific control to improved profits.

Dbcp Toxicology And Regulation

The toxicological testing of DBCP revealed serious fault lines in the exercise of scientific control over pesticide risks. In 1959, FIFRA was amended to include nematicides. Although the effective date for DBCP registration under the law was pushed back several times, Dow and Shell researchers knew their work would be pivotal in obtaining federal approval. By 1959, at least three toxicological studies conducted by Dow scientists or the University of California researchers contracted by Shell had shown that DBCP adversely affected the male reproductive organs in laboratory animals.

Scientists at both companies knew that these kinds of results in animals could mean danger for people exposed to the chemical; so did federal officials, who asked for more information on testicular damage and stronger warning label than the companies had proposed. Concerned with the potential effect of the stronger warning on profits, Shell pushed for – and regulators granted – an opportunity to counter animal toxicology with data supposedly demonstrating a "history of safe use" in manufacturing plants and agricultural settings. This approach ignored the fundamental premise of toxicology that animal studies provided a proxy for human health effects and instead insisted that human bodies were not subjects to the same risks as the monkeys, rats, guinea pigs, and rabbits in researchers' laboratories. More importantly, researchers did not examine exposed workers for testicular or related health effects. Nevertheless, company scientists excised earlier expressions of doubt or precaution, resulting in an interpretation that insisted that DBCP presented no special health hazards.

In March 1964, the USDA registered Nemagon and Fumazone, signaling the success of Dow and Shell in convincing the regulatory agencies to accept their version of DBCP toxicity. Despite initial concerns, regulators had yielded to the companies' characterization of it as safe for human use and approved mild warning language that contained no mention of testicular or any other chronic risk.

Conclusion

Dow and Shell did not live up to the industry's promise of scientifically impartial testing and warning. The companies marketed DBCP in scientific terms although the compound had not yet been thoroughly tested for safety, attaching to it the implicit claim of (relative) safety stemming from the voiced industry commitment to ascertaining safety before making a chemical commercially available. In reconciling the exigencies of their context of employment with the demands of a supposedly impartial science, scientists made choices that ultimately violated the tenets of toxicological inquiry and obscured DBCP's dangers. They did so, however, in a narrative that used the language and assumed the authority of science, by providing data and interpretation on a "history of safe use" of the chemical. Their actions ultimately set the stage for sterility among male production and agricultural workers that would be uncovered only in the late 1970s.

Tuberculosis Germs at Work: Infection, the Labour Movement and the British Workplace, c1900-1960

Arthur McIvor
University of Strathclyde, Glasgow, UK

In the UK, the first half of the twentieth century witnessed a fundamental shift in thinking about the aetiology of tuberculosis (TB) in one important respect that has been rather neglected in the literature. In the late nineteenth century the dominant view located TB as an infectious disease linked to hereditary dispositions, poor hygiene, diet and poverty, with urban living conditions – especially overcrowding - contributing significantly to its spread. By mid-twentieth century, TB was recognised to also be an occupational disease through the synergies with silica dust inhalation whilst at work and in its own right for health workers and others, who through the course of their employment came into contact with carriers of the disease. Thus, TB was effectively regarded as an occupational disease in a specified and limited fashion at least from the mid-1920s where it existed in conjunction with pneumoconiosis (initially silicosis in selected trades, but extended over time, for example, to include asbestosis and TB in 1931, and coal workers' pneumoconiosis and TB in 1942). After a long campaign, TB was also included in March 1951 as a prescribed occupational disease for health workers under the National Insurance (Industrial Injuries) Act (1946) which had superseded the workmen's compensation system. The latter scheduling of TB was innovative and created a precedent because no other disease prevalent in the general population in the UK had ever been defined officially as an occupational disease. The distinction was important because it gave a large group of relatively poorly paid health workers – including nurses – access to improved benefits.

Why did this occur? My research explores the evolving challenges to the prevailing medical orthodoxy regarding the aetiology of TB through the first half of the 20th century and examines, in particular, the role played by the trade unions and the labour movement in the process of redefining the significance of the workplace in the TB story. It draws upon the papers of the Trades Union Congress (UK), the Scottish Trade Union Congress and some other organisations, including the coal miners' unions and the Glasgow and District Trades Council.

The argument engages with the literature on the role of trade unions in occupational health, including the work of Long, Melling, and Bowden and Tweedale, amongst others.[1] The interpretation developed here, based on the evidence surveyed, is that the labour movement was much more proactive on tuberculosis than the literature indicates. The TUC was a pivotal player in the campaign to get TB scheduled as an industrial disease, whilst the Scottish TUC, local Trades Councils and individual unions were active both in relation to TB as a public health and an occupational health issue.

Using medical evidence generated by TB doctors and medical investigators like Alice Stewart, the labour movement campaigned on a number of fronts. From the 1920s, TB incidence was linked to occupation in a number of ways: including jobs with the lowest socio-economic status (such as casual labouring and clothing sweatshops); jobs where the site of production facilitated the spread of infection (including where relatively well paid craft workers were clustered together in light work as in footwear manufacture and printing) and employment where there was direct contact with known TB carriers / patients, as in the health services, asylums and prisons. The coal mining unions, led by the South Wales Miners Federation, campaigned to get the linkage between silicosis and tuberculosis recognised – and though not uncontested this "synergy" was accepted for compensation purposes (in the co-called 'Middleton formula') by 1927.[2] The TUC and the STUC also spearheaded the campaign in the 1940s to get TB officially scheduled as a prescribed occupational disease, marshalling lay epidemiology and medical surveys, such as the Royal College of Physicians 1948 investigation that quantified higher infection propensity amongst nurses. The enhanced bargaining power of labour in the general context of the Second World War and its aftermath – with the Labour Party landslide electoral victory – provided a favourable political, social and economic milieu for this unprecedented reform.

The labour movement in Scotland, where TB rates were particularly high, was especially active. The Scottish TUC applied pressure on the Scottish Department of Health and local authorities to radically improve preventative measures and compensation, including medical surveillance through mass x-rays, vaccination and campaigns against the infection hazards of overcrowded "slum workplaces" as well as "slum housing." In this the local Trades Councils (conglomerations of trade unions within a particular town or city) played a pivotal role, with the Glasgow Trades Council amongst the most active in the anti-TB campaign. The latter had an interest in TB within the community that dated back to the 1900s and a Standing Committee by the 1950s that initiated influential enquiries into incidence and the efficacy of medical screening for TB in the area. Together with other progressive groups, the latter contributed to the 1957 "mass assault" on TB in Glasgow, when almost the entire Glasgow population was screened by a fleet of mobile x-ray vans.

This case study then reiterates the porous nature of public health and occupational health and the intersections between the two, whilst providing further support for the view that the negative portrayal of the trade unions in public and environmental health policy in the literature merits some reconsideration. One editorial in 1957 in the journal Occupational Medicine read: "Trade unionists nowadays are extremely health-conscious."[3] Perhaps the view of one trade union delegate that the Trades Union Congress was 'the custodian of the health and welfare of the working class' was more than just empty rhetoric after all.[4]

I am particularly grateful to my colleague Ronnie Johnston for providing comments on an earlier draft of the longer paper presented at the conference on which this expanded abstract is based.

REFERENCES

[1] See Long V.The Rise and Fall of the Healthy Factory: The Politics of Industrial Health in Britain, 1914-60. Basingstoke: Palgrave Macmillan: 2011, for the most in-depth investigation of the role of the British Trades Union Congress in occupational health; Melling J. *The Risks of Working and the Risks of Not Working: Trade Unions, Employers and Responses to the Risk of Occupational Illness in British Industry, c1890-1940s*. ESRC Centre for Analysis of Risk and Regulation Discussion Paper 12, 2003,14-34; Bowden S and Tweedale G. Mondays without Dread: The Trade Unions' Response to Byssinosis in the Lancashire Cotton Industry in the Twentieth Century. *Social History of Medicine*, 16, 2003, 79-96.

[2] Bufton M and Melling J. Coming up for Air: Experts, Employers and Workers in Campaigns to Compensate Silicosis Sufferers in Britain, 1918-39. *Social History of Medicine*, 18 (2005), 63-86; McIvor A and Johnston R. *Miners' Lung: A History of Dust Disease in British Coal Mining*. Ashgate; Aldershot; 2007.

[3] *Occupational Medicine*, July 1957, no 7, 65.

[4] TUC Annual Report, 1955, 377. The comment was made by C. Plant, a Civil Service TB Sanatorium officer and representative of the Inland Revenue Staff Federation.

The Birth of the Italian Workers' Compensation Authority and its Contribution to Improving Health Conditions of Workers and General Population

Giuseppe Bonifaci[1], Michele A. Riva[2], Claudia Sferra[1], Matteo Marchesi[3], Vittorio A. Sironi[2]

[1] *Italian Workers' Compensation Authority (INAIL), Rome, Italy*

[2] *Research Centre on the History of Biomedical Thought, University of Milano Bicocca, Milan, Italy*
[3] *Dept of Experimental Medicine, University of Milano Bicocca, Milan, Italy*

After the conclusion of its unification in 1870, Italy had to make its legislation uniform all over the regions of the new State. The first proposed law on work accident insurance was introduced by Pietro Pericoli (1822-1889) in 1877, but it was initially criticized by the liberal forces due to potential financial risks for the State.[1] Only in 1883 the Italian Parliament enacted a law on "optional" work accident insurance, which leaded to the creation of a National Accident Fund, named "Cassa Nazionale di Assicurazione per gli Infortuni degli operai sul Lavoro" (CNAIL). The purpose was encouraging the employers to insure their workers, especially in view of low premium rates that were practiced. However this insurance, as well as preventive and security measures, were seen as a great economic burden for industries. Hence only a few employees were insured.[2] In 1884 Germany was the first country to introduce the compulsory work accident insurance in its legislation. In that period, Germany was militarily allied with Italy and it was considered as a model for all the legislative reforms, mainly in the welfare system. So, in 1898 the Italian Parliament enacted a law introducing the compulsory work accident insurance and extending the compensation even if the fault was attributed to the employee.[1] Despite these innovations, the coverage was limited to a few categories – rural workers were not insured – and only partial compensation was provided to the employees. In addition, this law did not identify a single insurance company: both public and private organizations could provide insurance. At the beginning of the 20th century, further extension of the social protection to specific worker categories was introduced in Italian legislation. These laws were expression of the new political climate, when several reforms were made to modernize the industrial sector of the country.[3] In that period, CNAIL increased its activities by opening outpatient clinics in all the largest Italian cities. Medical aid was closer to the injured workers and also increasingly effective. In 1913 CNAIL opened a clinic for first aid to injured workers in Libya (Italian colony at that period) and struck an agreement with hospitals in Tripoli and Bengasi for inpatient treatment.[4] Meanwhile, in August 1917, the Italian Parliament extended compulsory insurance also to rural workers. In the following years, a network of clinics, differently equipped but all with tools for emergency surgery, was established by the CNAIL in the whole country and first hospitals for injured workers were founded.

From 1922 until 1943, Fascism involved a corporatist political system in which the economy was collectively managed by employers, workers and state officials through formal mechanisms at national level.[3] So, private organizations were forbidden to provide work accident insurance and in 1933 the CNAIL was unified with other small public funds in a single establishment, the Istituto Nazionale Fascista per l'Assicurazione contro gli Infortuni sul Lavoro (INFAIL). In the same years, six occupational diseases (Ankylostomiasis; lead, mercury, carbon disulfide, phosphorus and benzene poisonings) were recognized by Italian legislation and therefore compensated.[3] After the fall of Fascism, INFAIL was renamed Istituto Nazionale per l'Assicurazione contro gli Infortuni sul Lavoro (INAIL, Italian Workers' Compensation Authority). During the post-war recovery, the Italian economic growth led to an increase in the industrial production and consequently in work accidents. INAIL had to provide a fully dedicated system to the care of injuries at workplace and occupational diseases. For this reason, it founded several hospitals and outpatient clinics. In the fifties, INAIL had 297 outpatient clinics, 8 hospitals fully dedicated to work traumas and named "Centri Ortopedici-Traumatologici" (CTO, Orthopedic Traumatic Centers) with 1,528 beds in the whole country (Milan, Bologna, Rome, Bari, Iglesias, Trento and Palermo).

Two hospitals were under construction (Naples: 206 beds; Padua: 275 beds) and two hospitals were designed (Florence and Turin). Moreover INAIL properties included 2 centers for re-education (Milan and Palermo), 6 convalescent homes, 7 research centers on occupational diseases, 16 first aid locations, 1 center for paraplegics "Villa Marina" in Ostia, near Rome. Finally, 38 trauma wards (1700 beds) were managed by INAIL in hospitals not belonging to the Authority.[4] The director of INAIL Paraplegics Center, Antonio Maglio (1912-1988), first used new techniques and methods for rehabilitation through sports in Italy, organizing a wheelchair fencing competition in 1957. After the great success in fencing, Maglio persuaded Sir Ludwig Guttmann (1899-1980), creator of the Stoke Mandeville Games (originally only for war veterans with spinal cord lesions) to organize an international event in the months following the Olympic Games in Rome. So, in September 1960 INAIL and "Italian National Olympic Committee" (CONI) organized the first International Paralympic Games in Rome with over 400 contestants. The Italian National Health System born in 1978, thus all health structures originally owned by INAIL were assigned to the Ministry of Health. Since then INAIL has been committed only in medical-legal activities. In August 2009 a Parliament enactment let INAIL provide directly healthcare in agreement with each region. Today, the mission of INAIL is a "completed and integrated protection of the worker" through prevention campaigns, direct treatment and rehabilitation of the injured workers, medico-legal assessment, evaluation of residual functional capacities and both social and occupational reintegration. In detail, this mission is fully achieved in the "Centro Protesi INAIL" (INAIL Prosthesis Centre), located in Vigorso di Budrio, near Bologna. Founded in 1961, the "Centro Protesi" is a centre of excellence, by constructing and applying personal orthopaedic prostheses not only to injured workers, but also to the general population, with rehabilitation and social reintegration purposes.

REFERENCES

Cataldi E. L'Istituto Nazionale per l'Assicurazione contro gli Infortuni sul lavoro: testimonianza di un secolo. Roma: Edizioni INAIL; 1983. Italian

Busacchi V. D'Antuono G. La medicina del lavoro nei suoi sviluppi storici. Roma: E. Cossidente; 1967. Italian

Carnevale F, Baldasseroni A. Mal da lavoro: storia della salute dei lavoratori. Roma: Editori Laterza; 1999. Italian

Moriniello A. Origine e sviluppo della tutela dei lavoratori contro le malattie professionali. Milano: Tipolitografia INAIL; 1959. Italian

The history of the workers´ compensation in Sweden

Sara Stendahl[1], Kjell Torén[2]

[1]Department of Law, University of Gothenburg, Gothenburg, Sweden;
[2]Section of Occupational and environmental medicine, University of Gothenburg, Gothenburg, Sweden

The first workers' compensation law came into effect in 1901 in Sweden – late compared to other industrialized countries. The first bill proposed in the Swedish parliament in 1881 reflected the German workers´ compensation system. This and several bills that followed, however, was rejected by parliament. At that time the compensation system issues was the business of liberal politicians. The labor party had no seats in the parliament. Sweden was an agrarian country at the time, and the resistance to pass these bills reflected a coalition between well-to-do farmers and rural industrialists. The bill that passed in 1901 was based on no-fault principle, the qualifying period was 60 days and the daily allowance was 30% of the salary of an ordinary worker. This was one of the least generous compensation laws in western Europe and the single labor party member of the parliament, Hjalmar Branting, voted against it expressing that this bill shamed Sweden.

The law was out of date already when it came into effect. During this period Norway left the union with Sweden 1905, the labor party and the labor unions increase their societal influence and in 1911 the first election was held with universal suffrage (only for men). This resulted in a changed power balance in the parliament, as the right wing parties gained less influence.

The low compensation levels of the workers´ compensation prompted the creation of a number of local mutual insurance schemes between labor unions and employers. This resulted in pressure from employers to modernize the workers´ compensation law. The liberal government decided in 1910 to appoint a new committee with the mission to thoroughly analyse to social security system (or the absence of such system) and to propose new bills. Chair was Anders Lindstedt, and two of the participating members were Hjalmar Branting and Sven Palme. This committee proposed in 1915 (during World War I) a quite generous (for its time) law with mandatory rule for all employers to insure their employees the daily allowance was proportional to the income, there was no qualifying period and the law also comprised occupational diseases. The bill passed in 1916, however, the occupational diseases had been deleted and there was an addition of four qualifying days. Hence, the compensation covered only accidents, and only in 1929 were occupational diseases covered by the legislation. The law applied only to listed diseases or exposures and this schedule was valid until 1976.

In 1976, the Swedish parliament, with the support of all parties, passed a new occupational compensation law. This was a unique law, as it stated that all diseases and accidents should be regarded as occupational "if there is not considerable evidence against an association." With this Act Sweden abandoned the system of listed occupational diseases and transitioned to a system where in principle all diseases could be certified as occupational. The system required certification, preferably but not necessarily, from a physician, outlining the scientific evidence for the association between the disease or condition and the occupational exposure. The Swedish medical profession was unprepared for this task: civil servants in regional social insurance offices soon assumed the task of reaching conclusions regarding causal associations, often supporting such associations. By late 1980s, 90% of all reported diseases were certified based on an underlying opinion that the burden of proof should not be worn by the individual but by society. In 1993, the parliament passed a new bill, now outlining a more restrictive scheme. This restrictive bill was reflecting the economic crisis that was very fulminant in Sweden in the beginning of 1990s.

This new law was heavily criticised and in 2002 a new bill was proposed. In that was stated that all diseases should be regarded as occupational diseases if "predominant evidence" is in favour of an association. The practice that was established was that "predominant evidence" means that the attributable fraction should exceed 50%, meaning that the relative risk should be greater than two.

References

Barth PS, Hunt HA. *Workers' compensation and work-related illnesses and diseases.* MIT Press, Cambridge, England, 1980

Englund, K. Arbetarförsäkringsfrågan i svensk politik 1884-1901. Studia historica Upsaliensia 82, Uppsala, 1976 [In Swedish].

Harrington JM, Newman Taylor AJ, Coggon D. Industrial injuries compensation. Br J Ind Med 1991;48:577-578.

Measuring Disability: Evaluating the Corporal Damage in Occupational Accident Victims and the Development of Occupational Health in Spain, 1900-1936

José Martinez-Perez, Mercedes Del Cura
Unit for the History of Science
Faculty of Medicine of Albacete
University of Castilla-La Mancha, Spain

This work has been possible thanks to the funding awarded by the Consejeria of Education and Science of the Junta de Comunidades de Castilla-La Mancha (Ref. PAI05-009).

Introduction

At the end of the 19th century a series of important legislation aimed at regulating various aspects related to occupational accidents was passed in Spain, in conjunction with what was happening in Europe.[1] One of the milestones of this legislation was the Occupational Accidents Law of January 30th 1900 (OAL-1900). This illustrated that the State was interested in dealing with a matter that was becoming a social problem. The new laws, not only sought to lessen the economic and human damage that death or disability caused to the workers and their families, but were also designed to tackle the negative consequences that occupational accidents had on something that was deemed to be key to functioning of the nation, that is maintaining and increasing production.

If occupational accidents were becoming a problem, the Medicine was meant to play an important role to solve it. The OAL-1900 stipulated that employers were not only obliged to provide medical care for the victims and set up a system to pay compensation to the workers affected. It meant that doctors found themselves in an important strategic position as they were entrusted with the task of evaluating the injuries.[2]

For the aims of this work we are interested in highlighting the way in which this task, that in which the doctors determined the degree of disability resulting from the injuries caused by the accident, helped the early specialists to become experts in understanding and dealing with disability. This work also aims to illustrate how the discourse that the new specialists generated regarding this matter had an influence on the social identity of those affected by the physical impairments.

The Rise Of A New Discourse About Disability

To see how a medical discourse on these problems was developing in Spain we have to look at the Royal National Academy of Medicine (RNAM). This institution gathered information on difficult cases and prepared reports that had to be conclusive in order to resolve lawsuits. The first case on which the RNAM had to rule was recorded on 1903 (Dossier 101. Portfolio 211, Years 1902-1903. Library of the Royal National Academy of Medicine). An object fell onto the right foot of a port stevedore (June 13th 1901), and the injury did not heal well. Months later, the doctor that had been treating the victim decided he was recovered and could go back to his job (April 19, 1902). However the worker claimed that he could not work because "his foot got tired." The doctor responsible for the final decision regarding the condition of the worker said that the worker´s opinion could not be "determined exactly" and so wanted other doctors to intervene to determine the situation. One month later, one of the new experts deemed the worker fit for work, but the other two thought that the victim was not "in a suitable condition to undertake his usual work" and that he had been left "useless for the work he did." This early case illustrates some of the problems that we are interested in. Firstly, it is clear that the first demands that the OAL-1900 made on doctors put them in a difficult position. Their role as experts meant that they had to decide on matters which they did not always feel able to make a conclusive decision due to a complete lack of information of the facts, or to the technical limitations of the doctor involved or those of medicine itself to do what was asked.

A second issue was one that arose because several experts were involved. The contradictory decisions emphasised the limitations of medicine to provide a categorical answer and a single front to the questions raised and so questioned the ability of the doctors to meet the expectations given to them by the new law.

Lastly, the doctors' answers, by having to decide whether what the workers claimed about their health was true, helped to highlight the possibility that the worker victims of occupational accidents were trying to feign a physical or functional impairment in order to benefit from the compensations and advantages of the OAL-1900.

But, as another cases dealt with by the RNAM illustrates, the application of the OAL-1900, and the medical discourse which this was contributing to elaborate, had another consequences for the victims of an accident at the workplace. In one of the first cases on the RNAM was consulted, it was introduced the problem of how to manage the situation in which the workers had "subjective symptoms and easy to feign" and the "scientific data" was "insufficient to determine whether or not there was in fact some kind of suffering." The solution given for the experts was asking the worker "if he had any certificates from the workshop where he applied his trade."[3]

From our point of view, this case illustrates another aspect of the process that we are studying: the fact that the limitations of Medicine to establish the existence and extent of certain injuries were having undesired effects on the workers. The experts, far from not passing a judgement on these situations, tried to make decisions in a way that helped cast the shadow of fraud on the occupational accident victims. In these cases, the affected worker was obliged to provide data on his moral integrity which helped give the experts the impression that they were honest workers and thus lead them to believe that they were not feigning their complaints. So, the worker's behaviour became a part of the process aimed at settling these lawsuits.

Conclusions

The OAL-1900, by obliging any worker who wished to take advantage of the benefits of the law to have orthodox medical treatment and be examined by medical experts, resulted in disability becoming focused on corporal and/or mental abnormality. In this way, the discourse that we are studying considerably helped the development of a kind of approach to disabilities which has been named "medical model" of disability by the disabled activist. This approach leads to a way of understanding disability that sees its solution in medical knowledge. As a result, this model has been considered an obstacle for the way of seeing the problem of disability that has been defined as a "social model." This way of seeing the problem does not deny the significance of physical disability in the lives of the disabled, but, unlike the "medical model," focuses on the numerous obstacles—economic, social and cultural...that have built up around them.[4]

There is no doubt that the OAL-1900 helped to improve the situation of workers and their families. However, the application of the law also meant that difficult situations arose which had serious consequences for those had directly affected by the accidents. The discrepancies between the various decisions of the experts in charge of evaluating the workers' injuries did little to reinforce the image that medicine was trying to transmit as a science of absolute and indisputable truths. The doctors, nevertheless, tried to comply with the law by incorporating aspects that in fact took them away from the objectivity that was expected of them. Taking into account such aspects as the worker´s good behaviour meant applying in the decision making such subjective criteria that brought the testimonies given by the accident victims under suspicion.

This last point, the possibility that some accident victims might feign the extent of their injuries, was detrimental to the social image of those affected by anatomical or functional impairments. At a time when society had agreed to compensate the victims of occupational accidents, the possibility that people who might be classified "invalids" and who were not really disabled were benefiting from this was not at all beneficial for other people with impairments. If we add this to the fact that the law also helped to reinforce the link between disability and the ability to work, which enhanced the image of someone affected as being unable to fully contribute to the economy, it illustrates how the OAL-1900 also helped to develop an image of those affected as being dependent and unproductive.

References
[1] Soto Carmona A. *La higiene, la seguridad y los accidentes del trabajo. España (1874-1936)*. Civitas. Revista Española del Derecho del Trabajo. 1985; 23: 389-423. Spanish.
[2] Rodriguez Ocaña E. Industrielle Gesundheitsgefährdung und Medizin in Spanien, 1850-1936. Eine Annäherung an den medizinischen Diskurs. In: Milles D, ed., *Gesundheitsrisiken, Industriegesellschaft und soziale Sicherungen in der Geschichte*. Bremerhaven: Wirtschaftsverlag NW - Verlag für neue Wissenschaft GmbH; 2002. p. 419-440.
[3] *De la segunda Comisión de Medicina forense, en un expediente sobre accidentes del trabajo*. Anales de la Real Academia Nacional de Medicina. 1904; 24: 223-226. Spanish.
[4] Barnes C, Mercer G, Shakespeare T. *Exploring Disability. A Sociological Introduction*. Cambridge: Polity Press; 2002.

The Trades Union Congress and the Politics of Industrial Health in Britain, 1920-1960

Vicky Long
University of Strathclyde, Glasgow, Scotland, UK

Has the trade union movement historically failed to protect workers' health?[1] In his 1985 edited volume on the history of occupational health, Paul Weindling argued that trade unions had tended to prioritize pay and compensation at the expense of health issues.[2] The development and delivery of industrial health provisions was, however, contingent upon the outcome of negotiations between different interest groups. Drawing upon research undertaken on the archives of the Trades Union Congress (hereafter TUC), employer organizations, medical associations, personnel organizations and government records, this abstract outlines the steps taken nationally by the TUC to improve the health of industrial workers and explores why it was not more successful in the field of industrial health.

Established in 1868 to coordinate action amongst trade unions in England and Wales, the TUC had little autonomous power. It could only implement policy decisions after securing the consent of its affiliated unions and did not have the financial resources to establish its own large-scale research or treatment facilities. Despite these limitations, the TUC was an enthusiastic advocate of industrial health services. It adopted a variety of approaches in its attempts to enact its health promotion objectives in tandem with and as a natural adjunct to its work to extend the scheduling of industrial diseases under compensation legislation. In the interwar years, the TUC found itself hampered by a culture which gave precedence to professional expertise, enabling critics to undermine TUC campaigns on health care issues. An unfavorable economic climate drove down trade union membership, deterred employer investment in workplace facilities and curtailed state intervention in health care. The TUC attempted to circumvent these barriers in a number of ways, appointing Sir Thomas Legge, the former Senior Medical Factory Inspector, as its first Medical Advisor in 1930; Legge's expertise in industrial health ensured that TUC policy on health issues received greater attention. Throughout this period, the TUC was a vocal critic of a medical system which, in its view, compensated and cured the sick but did little to prevent illness from occurring. In deputations to the government the TUC attacked the inadequacies of the 1911 National Health Insurance Act. It criticized a system in which the panel doctors who provided treatment had little knowledge of their patients' working conditions, where little incentive was provided to prevent workers falling sick and no statistics were gathered to monitor patterns of illness. The TUC campaigned to ensure healthier working conditions through new factory legislation in the face of employer intransigence, sending a number of deputations to the government over the fifteen year period between the introduction of the first factory bill in 1923 and the passing of the 1937 Factories Act.

The TUC also sought to influence medical training and practice. In 1936, it submitted evidence to the General Medical Council advocating alterations to the medical curriculum that would enable future doctors to be educated about health as well as illness. It collaborated with the British Medical Association, established a joint committee to discuss issues of mutual concern. The TUC and its affiliated unions experimented with a number of voluntary initiatives to improve workers' health; trade union funds, for example, helped maintain the Manor House Hospital which provided orthopaedic treatment to ameliorate the effects of industrial accidents and disease. The extensive financial support afforded to the hospital by trade unions belies the argument that trade unions were disinterested in health issues; what it does suggest is that there was a greater willingness to support projects which sought to remedy visible physical damage caused by injury or disease, rather than invest in preventive or mental health services. Employers' unwillingness to accept responsibility for workers' health prompted the TUC to advocate the establishment of a state-run national industrial health service. Increasingly, it expressed the concern that voluntary provisions could provide the government with an opportunity to avoid implementing legislation which would ensure improved conditions within all workplaces and comprehensive health services.

Although disappointed that industrial health services had been excluded from the National Health Service, inaugurated in 1948, the TUC remained confident that a national industrial health service would subsequently be established. In the postwar era, it was the most persistent advocate of a comprehensive state-run occupational health service which could prevent ill-health by monitoring workers' health and working environments, but was outmaneuvered by economic and political factors which lay outside its control. Rivalry between the ministries of Labour and Health pushed the government to investigate whether industrial health provisions should be curtailed to ensure the survival of the fledgling National Health Service. As only 2% of Britain's doctors and nurses were employed in industrial health services, it is perhaps not surprising that the ensuing report recommended that the government establish an advisory committee to coordinate developments in industrial health services with a view to expanding provisions.[3] These findings were accepted by the incumbent Labour government. The Conservative government, elected shortly afterwards, had no interest in developing services but was aware that openly stating their intention to do nothing could prove politically problematic. In 1954, the prospect of an imminent election, combined with relentless pressure from the TUC and the British Medical Association, impelled the Minister of Labour to propose a scheme to develop national occupational health services. At Cabinet, these proposals were rejected due to opposition from the Ministry of Health and concerns that an extension of occupational health services would be at odds with the government's policy of cutting costs. When the Conservative government's majority increased in the 1955 election, its interest in developing occupational health services evaporated. While the TUC continued to press for a comprehensive occupational health service, the Ministry of Labour repeatedly insisted that further investigation was required before a decisive course of action could be taken. Growing concern with industrial efficiency in an era of high employment aided and abetted this policy of procrastination, thwarting the TUC and helping the government to marginalize the issue of workers' health.

REFERENCES
[1] This paper stems from a Wellcome Trust-funded project, "The Politics and Practices of Health in Work in Britain, 1915-60," undertaken at the University of Warwick and managed by Professor Hilary Marland and Dr Mathew Thomson. For a detailed discussion of the findings from this project see Long V. *The Rise and Fall of the Healthy Factory: The Politics of Industrial Health in Britain, 1914-60*. Basingstoke: Palgrave Macmillan; 2010.
[2] Weindling P, editor. *The Social History of Occupational Health*. London: Croom Helm, 1985, p. 10.
[3] Report of a Committee of Enquiry on Industrial Health Services, Cmd 8170 (1951).

An Enslaved Population: The Work of Italian Military Internees (IMI) in Germany, 1943-1945

Porro Alessandro,[1] Falconi Bruno,[1] Cristini Carlo,[2] Lorusso Lorenzo,[3] Colombo Andrea,[4] Franchini Antonia Francesca[4]
[1] *Sezione di Scienze Umane e Medico Forensi. Dipartimento di Specialità Chirurgiche, Scienze Radiologiche e Medico Forensi. Università degli Studi di Brescia. Brescia. Italy*
[2] *Sezione di Psicologia. Dipartimento Materno Infantile e Tecnologie Biomediche. Università degli Studi di Brescia. Brescia, Italy*
[3] *U.O. di Neurologia, A.O. "Mellino Mellini". Chiari, Italy*
[4] *Dipartimento di Scienze Mediche. Università degli Studi di Milano. Milano, Italy*

After the armistice (September 8, 1943) the German troops occupied the most part of Italian territory. 600.000 Italian soldiers were deported in Germany (mostly from Greece, Balkans, Eastern Europe). With a document by VIII Corps (Greece) Commander (September 10, 1943, when Italian troops were unarmed), the Lieutenant General Mario Marghinotti (1887-?), indicates the destiny of Italian soldiers: "una strada quanto mai erta e dolorosa" (a steep and painful way). General Marghinotti would be a German POW (Prisoner Of War). Only honour and discipline remained to Italian soldiers, as opportunity of surviving. They were first considered POW, but Hitler denied their status in a short time, defining them Italian Military Internees (IMI: Italienischen Militaer Internirten, Internati Militari Italiani). So, the Geneva Convention didn't protect them. Internment (concentration) camps were distributed over the entire Reich's territory. IMI's life and work conditions were like those of an extermination camp, because the Italian soldiers were considered traitors. The work was hardest and daily rations very scarce. After the so called Salò Republic (Repubblica Sociale Italiana) establishment (the state Mussolini founded in Northern Italy in 1943), some of them joined its army (someone hoping to reach Italy and then to desert), but the majority of them preferred to stay in internment (concentration) camps. Mines, underground factories and installations were their principal work places. We can describe them with the word "slavery" (IMI were really slaves). A nazi war criminal described Dora (an underground factory where V2 were assembled): "the hell of concentration camps" (20.000 dead, 200 every day). Even when they worked in the country, they were often obliged to come back to Internment (concentration) camp, where hygiene and nutrition were scarce. In july, 1944 they became Civil Internee, but their real condition of life and work didn't change. In our paper we present some postcards sent by the internees to their families in Italy, dated from summer 1944. They show the frightful life and work conditions of these internees. Some postcards are propaganda postcards, created to persuade Italian civilians to cooperate with the German occupying troops. What kind of news could arrive in Italy from internment (concentration) camps? What splinter of truth? Most of Italian territory was occupied by German troops. All the communications were censored. The first postcard comes from STALAG VI D (Dortmund) a soldier writes: "Dear aunt rose… I feel all right." Dortmund Stalag was one of the worst camps. From STALAG IX C (Bad Sulza – Muehlhausen) "the health is good." But the truth comes from STALAG VI J (Krefeld – Fichtenheim). It was a STRAFLAGER, i.e., a punishment camp: "Supplies are running out… Send us wheat, pasta, beans…" Sometimes, the irony peeps out: an underlined phrase ("il mio mistiere [sic!] bello," my wonderful job) related to ore shovel, shows us the real condition of life and work. From STALAG XI B (Fallingbostel) and STALAG XI A (Altengrabow) comes out the homesickness. Eventually liberation comes (1945, april 13). From a diary by Ernesto Sarrantonio, the day after liberation (OFFLAG 83 – Wietzendorf): "14 aprile [1945]. Il sole splende ancora più bello di ieri. Siamo finalmente ritornati uomini! Non più numeri, non più un branco di pecore o di schiavi in mano agli aguzzini!" ("[1945,] april 14. The sun is shining. It's more beautiful than yesterday. We are men again. We are no more numbers, no more herd, no more slaves, no more in torturers' hands"). Some internees came back from Germany only in 1947, but all of them suffered psychological troubles. Only in the last twenty-year period historians dealt with this difficult subject. It was a not known Resistance against Nazis and fascists.

REFERENCES

Schreiber G. Die italienischen Militaer-internierten im deutschen Machtbereich 1943-1945. Verraten-verachtet-vergessen. Muenchen: Oldenbourg; 1990 (italian translation: I militari italiani internati nei campi di concentramento del terzo reich 1943-145. Roma: Stato Maggiore dell'Esercito. Ufficio storico; 1997).

Hammermann G. Zwangsarbeit fuer den Verbundeten: Die Arbeits- und Lebensbedingungen der italienischen Militaerinternierten in Deutschland 1943 -1945. Tuebingen: Niemeyer; 2002 (italian translation: Gli internati militari italiani in Germania 1943-145. Bologna. Il Mulino; 2004).

Avagliano M., Palmieri M. Gli internati militari italiani. Diari e lettere dai lager nazisti 1943-1945. Torino: Einaudi; 2009.

Chiesa P. Carissima famiglia... La Croce Rossa e le lettere dei prigionieri di guerra milanesi 1940-1946. Milano: Mursia; 2009.

Sarrantonio E. Ricordi della prigionia in Germania. Manuscript (private collection).

Sea Fevers: The Management of Infectious Disease at Sea in the British Merchant Fleet 1868-1967

Tim Carter

Norwegian Center for Maritime Medicine, University of Bergen, Bergen, Norway

In 1868 the British authorities sanctioned a single medical guide that was to be carried by all UK merchant ships. This was a novel step, with one authoritative guide replacing a number of publications with no official status. The earlier guides in the UK have yet to be investigated in detail although similar guides published in the USA have been studied.[1] The aim of the new "Ship Captain's Medical Guide" was to provide a sound framework for prevention, diagnosis and treatment of injuries and diseases arising at sea on vessels that did not carry a doctor that was fully compatible with the statutory list of ship medical stores. Because of its users it was written in straightforward language and emphasized the role of Nature as the healer with medical and nursing care assisting the process. A book of the same title is still a requirement for UK flagged ships and there have been 22 editions between 1868 and the present.[2]

Between 1868 and 1967 there were many changes in the understanding of the natural history of infectious diseases and their management; the evolving text of each edition of the Guide has been used to review these changes and how they were simplified to provide practical guidance to the officers on merchant ships. The pattern of infections changed with the sudden recurrence of old ones, such as plague in the 1890s, and the near elimination of others, such as smallpox, by improved prevention. The change from sail to steam altered the pattern of work aboard and shortening voyages. The introduction of radio enabled advice to be obtained in the event of a medical emergency, while at the end of the period helicopter evacuation from ships in coastal waters became possible.

At the time of the first edition current theories about infection distinguished between contagious diseases, such as smallpox and venereal infections and those associated with decay and local conditions – miasmatic diseases. This is reflected in early editions, which emphasize the use of disinfectants not to kill germs but to "purify." Germ theory begins to underlie preventive advice from 1885, first in relation to water borne diseases and those spread by faecal contamination. Thus typhus and typhoid were separated rather than both being seen as "continuing fevers." The Guide avoided the controversy about germ theory and only introduced new concepts only when they were well established and are relevant to the action that needs to be taken.[3]

The second major development in prevention that is reflected in the Guide is the role of arthropod vectors in disease transmission.[4] Malaria is linked to marshland until 1885 but between 1899 and 1912 the Anopheles mosquito moves from being a contributor to being the sole transmitter of the disease with precautions against mosquito bites as the main means of prevention. While malaria was a disease where UK was in the lead, USA scientists unraveled the role of the mosquito in yellow fever in 1900 but the Guide was a little slower to recognize this.

"It is a distinctly infectious disease and the infection is believed to be chiefly in the vomit;" 1912, "The sole agent for spreading the disease is the female mosquito of what is known as the Stegomyia or 'Tiger' species;" "...it is harmless until it has bitten a person suffering from yellow fever...."

Decisions of treatment depended on a diagnosis being made by an officer. The Guide aimed to equip officers for this task. Distinguishing signs of each infection were included, in tables from 1901 onwards. The use of the clinical thermometer as an aid to diagnosis received prolonged attention in the 1880s. Both its costs for ship operators and the ability of officers to read it were raised as arguments against its inclusion, but it was pointed out that reading a sextant was a far more difficult task than reading a thermometer it subsequently became a requirement. Cost was also an issue in relation to the use of colour plates in the Guide to show rashes; these were not included until 1952. Training in medical care and first aid to complement the advice in the Guide was developed from the 1890s.

In the 19th Century there were only effective treatments for two infections: quinine for malaria and mercury for syphilis. Treatment focused on symptom relief, isolation and good nursing, but within the limitations of crew quarters. The introduction of arsenicals to treat syphilis from 1910 led to new requirements for port medical investigation and care but it was not until sulphonamides and then antibiotics became available in the 1940s that care at sea moved to a phase of active treatment. Penicillin posed particular problems as early forms had to be mixed and given by injection; a skill that had to be taught to, often unwilling, officers.

The Ship Captain's Medical Guide provides a near unique resource for following the way in which a lay guide on health care developed in response to changes in knowledge. Its style also indicates the ways in which its medical authors thought that the treatment of infectious disease could and should be handled by those with limited medical skills in a setting where infection could threaten individuals; the crew generally and the safe operation of the ship, as well as causing problems with health officials when the ship docked. The health risks and care requirements in merchant seafarers have rarely been the subject of study, despite being a group with a complex pattern of risks and also being travellers liable to encounter exotic infections and carry them to new locations.[5]

The Guide also shows the strengths and weaknesses of the state sanctioning of a single source of reference, with continuing cost controls and the need to reflect current government policies in contentious areas such as the use of antibiotics and the precautions against venereal disease. The Guide's compatibility with statutory medical stores and its use in training and in standardising the dialogue when obtaining shore-based medical advice are rational strengths, but the inherent benefit of having an "authorised version" on the captain's shelf, traditionally next to the bible, as a source of definitive guidance which, if followed, would exonerate him from blame in the event of a fatal outcome cannot be over-estimated.

References

[1] Gordon E. Sailors Physicians: medical guides for merchant ships and whalers. 1774-1868. *J History of Medicine and Allied Sciences*, 1993; 48: 139-156.

[2] Leach H. *The Ship Captain's Medical Guide*. Simkin Marshall, London. 1st Edition 1868. Subsequent editions to 22nd The Stationery Office, London 1999. 2nd Edition available in facsimile on Google Books.

[3] Worboys, M. *Spreading Germs: Disease Theories and Medical Practie in Britain, 1865-1900*. Cambridge University Press, 2000

[4] Cox FEG (Editor). *The Wellcome Trust illustrated History of Tropical Diseases*. Wellcome, London 1996

[5] Carter T. *The Ship Captain's Medical Guide and the management of infectious disease at sea 1867-1967*. Dissertation, University of Greenwich, 2010

The Dawning of Accident Prevention In Milan: Workers, Trade Unions, Society, 1894-1896

Bruno Falconi,[1] Alessandro Porro,[1] Lorenzo Lorusso,[2] Andrea Colombo,[1] Antonia Francesca Franchini[3]

[1]Dipartimento di Specialità Chirurgiche, Scienze Radiologiche e Medico Forensi. Sezione di Scienze Umane e Medico Forensi. Università degli Studi di Brescia, Brescia, Italy

[2]Unità Operativa di Neurologia. Azienda Ospedaliera "Mellino Mellini" di Chiari, Chiari, Italy

[3]Dipartimento di Scienze Mediche. Università degli Studi di Milano, Milan, Italy

Milan was the main industrial city of Italian Kingdom, but it was a walled city, surrounded by another city, called Corpi Santi (Holy Bodies, with reference to the legend of the Magi, the three Wise Men). In 1873, Corpi Santi was incorporated, so that Milan could take advantage of a rural territory.

On this territory we'll find a textile print factory and a clinic: they will bring us into the main theme: the dawning of accident prevention. In the western neighborhood of the city, on the bank of Olona river, Ernesto De Angeli started up a textile print factory destined to became the main Italian textile print factory (Società Italiana per l'Industria dei Tessuti Stampati – De Angeli-Frua).

The Olona river, the cradle of Italian cotton industry, is mentioned by history of occupational health (Casati's studies concerning osteomalacy).

Ernesto De Angeli (1849-1907) founded the industrial association in Milan, and became Senator too.

At the end of XIXth century, industrial accidents were a problem to be studied; they were a problem to be solved.

International Congresses devoted to study industrial accidents and social assurances were held: the third of them took place at Milan in 1894, from the 1st to the 6th of October.

747 delegates debated the themes. They came from Italy (367), France (167), Germany (98), Switzerland (27), Austria-Hungary (23), Belgium (20), the Netherlands (20), Russian Empire (8), United Kingdom (7), USA (3), Spain (2), Brazil (1), Denmark (1), Norway (1), Portugal (1), Sweden (1).

Various themes were discussed: among them we can remind:

social and accident insurance

This theme was discussed and two positions were confronting: the voluntary, free insurance and the insurance required by law.

prevention of industrial accidents

The problem was analyzed from every side: we can remind general and particular means applied to mining industry; we can also remind individual protection devices as protective glasses or masks, and so on.

children, women and work

We remind socialist Anna Kuliscioff (between1853/57-1925).

With her speech, she proposed a strict control: for example, work conditions in mining industry were dangerous and painful.

Lawmaking

This aspect of preventing industrial accidents was discussed too.

The congress underlined: the need to plan and to carry out medical actions to reduce industrial accidents; the need to promote medical organizations; the need to open emergency surgical services devoted to treat injured persons.

The German example was proposed by Dr. von Boediker, President of the Imperial Insurance Office.

The insurance affected the treatment of injured workers positively. In 1895 Milanese Trade Unions deal with industrial accidents: a Congress devoted to study industrial accidents was held, from the 17th to the 19th of March. 170 associations or delegates were present, mostly from Lombardy and Emilia-Romagna. For the first time trade unions, working class debated industrial accidents.

We can remind also the presence of Senator De Angeli. For the first time, Ersilia Bronzini Majno (1859-1933), the founder of Women National Union came into contact with women's work and industrial accidents. The argument of her speech was: women's work regulation.

Other women delegates who debated this theme were (among the others): Annetta Ferla (League for women's interests), founder of Italian Workers Party (then Socialist Party); Giuditta Brambilla (Women's federation), from Milanese Trade union; Modesta Calcagni Rossi (Women's general association).

A medical association devoted to injured persons was opened in 1896. Senator De Angeli was president of the association from 1899 to 1907.

An emergency surgical service was opened in the northern (industrial) neighborhood of the city (7, Sarpi street). This was the sanitary staff: a Director (MD), a Vice-director (MD), chief of forensic service, three surgeons (MD), a physical therapist (MD), an ophthalmologist (MD), a neurologist (MD), two internists (MD), eleven doctors (MD), a chief nurse (male).

The relevance of medical Association's activity can be shown by its technical apparatuses and aids. For example, a first aid kit to be available in every factory and easily usable was produced. So, a first aid kit for the sanitary staff of the Medical Association was constructed too. The example was given by surgical and obstetrical ones. In 1898, in May the army took possession of the city of Milan: people built barricades; the army killed hundreds of people. The first wounded was cured at 7, Sarpi street. Association surgeons attended many wounded people in those days. Sarpi street clinic had a diversified surgical survey (neurosurgery, traumatology, plastic surgery, general surgery).

In conclusion, at the end of XIXth century, due to the working class and owners associations, in Milan prevention of industrial accidents (and medical cure of injured) was made possible.

References

Congrès international des Accidents du Travail et des Assurances Sociales. Troisième session tenue à Milan du 1er au 6 octobre 1894. Tome premier. Rapports. Milan: Imprimerie Henri Reggiani; 1894.

Congrès international des Accidents du Travail et des Assurances Sociales. Troisième session tenue à Milan du 1er au 6 octobre 1894. Tome second. Procès-verbaux des séances et communications présentées au congrès. Milan: Imprimerie Henri Reggiani; 1895.

Camera del Lavoro di Milano. Resoconto del Congresso sugl'infortuni del lavoro in rapporto all'igiene, al lavoro delle donne e dei fanciulli ed all'istruzione obbligatoria tenutosi in Milano nei giorni 17, 18 e 19 marzo 1895. Milano: Tipografia degli Operai; 1895.

Milano nel 1906. Milano: Tipografia Umberto Allegretti; 1906.

Rossi LE, Milano benefica e previdente. Cenni storici e statistici sulle istituzioni di beneficenza e di previdenza. Milano: Tipografia Francesco Marcolli; 1906.

L'Associazione per l'Assistenza Medica negli Infortuni del Lavoro di Milano (1896-1908). Milano: Stucchi e Ceretti; [1909].

The Fight Against Lead Poisoning in the Paint Industry: A Comparison of the French and American Experiences, 1900 - 1940

Judith Rainhorn

Université Lille-Nord de France / Institut universitaire de France, Lille, France

The aim of this paper is to compare two historical experiences on the issue of occupational health, in order to understand differences and similarities. Comparing the working conditions in France and the United States in terms of health and the risks of industrial poisoning allows me to: (i) discuss the often simplistic opposition between national "models" to be called into question (French prohibition vs. American dissuasion approach to occupational health); (ii) take occupational health out of the traditional binary conflict, capital/labor, that has long been a part of discussions about Labor history; (iii) reassess the issue of decisional levels with respect to legislation and social reform (national or federal/local).

Background

White lead had been clearly identified as a harmful agent in the paint industry, responsible for workers and painters intoxication in plants and painting sites. Its use nevertheless increased dramatically during the 19th century in main industrialized countries, thanks to its intense whiteness, well-covering and bad weather-proof power, making lead poisoning one of the most wide spread occupational diseases in both France and the US. On both sides of the Atlantic, scholars have emphasized the role of lead poisoning in revealing occupational health as a major public and political issue during the 20th century.[1]

Material and methods

This paper aims to investigate and compare actors, processes and chronological trends through two historical experiences (France and the US) on the issue of occupational lead poisoning in the paint industry in the early 20th century. It is based on primary material gathered both in France and the US, as periodicals and papers, medical surveys conducted at a plant or state level (particularly Alice Hamilton's papers), trade unions and hospital archives, and parliamentary debates.

I aim to examine different decision-making actors and scales, the role of the State (national in France / federal and local in the US), of doctors and social workers, of radicalism and unions, and of public debate, in order to assess the disclosure and process of giving up white lead paint in both countries, in a comparative perspective.

Results

1. In France, painters were first to be subject to protective measures, effected at the local and national levels at the very beginning of the 20th century: local laws (1900, 1902), a national decree (July 1902), and the 1903 proposition by the French Parliament of a law that would totally prohibit the use of white lead in all painting projects, which finally passed in 1909. At that time, no legislation was taken in the US, and Alice Hamilton visiting these plants described workers transporting shovels and wheelbarrows full of white lead powder through air permeated with white lead dust, without the benefit of protective clothing.

2. Compared to the vigorous campaing in the French press, the New York Times and the Brooklyn Eagle confirmed our impression of the lack of public awareness and interest in the issue of industrial poisoning before WW1. The trade unions, nor in France, neither in the US, were not leading the mobilization. In my opinion, the victory against lead paint in France was the result of a multiform mobilization of diverse social and political spheres, associating doctors, legislators, workers and members of the progressive reform circles. Reconstituting this mobilization also allows the importance of the local scale and the individual actor in the historical process to be understood. We can emphasize the role of Abel Craissac—former house painter himself and treasurer of the house painter trade union in Paris. He was fundamental in establishing the anti-white lead discourse within the French trade unions, for which he played an obvious role of trompe-l'œil.[2] In the US, the well-known Alice Hamilton played in some extent a similar role. Her work long remained

pioneering research.

3. In France, legal measures and regulations about health and safety were adopted at a quite slow pace in the first years of the 20th century: it means the very slow penetration of the State into the private relationships that govern labor and the closed space of the company. A prohibition process was begun: the law envisioned the suppression of white lead in 1915, but was never implemented because of the War. The early mobilization before the war probably facilitated the passage of the law of 1919, which created the compensation system for occupational diseases and put lead poisoning among the diseases at the top of the list. The ILO rapidly made the issue of white lead the subject of an international convention (1922). It seems relatively clear that France was a driving force in favor of prohibiting white lead. In the United States, the rapid turnover of industrial workers—with a huge proportion of recent European immigrants—disguised the importance of occupational diseases for a long time in a fully expanding economy. For this reason, in the 1910s and the 1920s, by showing that American factories had higher morbidity and mortality rates due to lead poisoning than European factories, Alice Hamilton gradually weakened the "Progressive era" myth of the superiority of American industry. Still, she barely changed the opinions of the general public. Thus, Alice Hamilton's work had an impact mostly on the reform movement in Chicago, who pushed the state legislators to action and in 1911, Illinois voted the first Workmen's Compensation Law. This local scale policy making did not employ prohibitionist logic, which would have forbidden toxic products, but rather financial dissuasion, with the financial stakes of insurance premiums. Henceforth, lead paint was almost progressively abandoned in the country: the sales of lead paint were divided in half in 6 years [between 1928 and 1934]. From 1913 to 1920, most of the American states adopted compensation legislation. Step by step, through economic and financial dissuasion, the risk of industrial poisoning was reduced for the workers in most paint factories and workshops.

Conclusion

This paper emphasizes the two different national ways to the same achievement: the decline of lead paint during the interwar period, resulting from different actors and processes. Based on two political, industrial and cultural contexts, this comparison enables to reassess the traditional opposition between policies of prohibition (France) and deterrence (US), between political, legal and economic weapons in fighting occupational diseases. It sheds light on the numerous transfers of scientific knowledge and social mobilizations on both sides of the Atlantic ocean.

REFERENCES

[1] Rosner D, Markowitz G. Dying for Work. Bloomington : Midland Books. Indiana University Press; 1987. C. Warren, *Brush with death. A social history of lead poisoning*. Saint-Louis: John Hopkins University Press; 2000. Rosental PA, Buzzi S, Devinck JC. *La santé au travail*. Paris: Repères; 2006.

[2] Rainhorn J. Le mouvement ouvrier contre la peinture au plomb: stratégie syndicale, expérience locale et transgression du discours dominant au début du XXe siècle. *Politix*. 2010; 91 (9-26).

The Struggle for Lead Poisoning Recognition in the Workplace in France: The 1970s Turning Point

Laure Pitti

University Paris 8/CRESPPA-CSU, Paris, France

The present paper deals with the issue of lead poisoning recognition in the workplace in France during the second half of the 20th century. Even though lead poisoning was the first occupational disease to be legally recognized in France as from 1919, some factories largely continued to produce lead until the 1970s, regardless of workers' health issues. This is the case of Peñarroya, on which this paper will focus. In the 1960s this company was the first lead producer in Europe and one of the three main lead producers in the world. It owned several mines and factories mainly based in Europe and North Africa and employed a large number of colonial and post-colonial migrant workers in its European plants as from the 1950s.

This paper sets out a three-part approach to study how and why lead poisoning became an important issue in the 1970s. First of all, it will focus on the progress of international medical knowledge as from the 1960s, especially on the biological approach of lead poisoning. Secondly, it will demonstrate how in France, this new step in medical knowledge was used and partly shaped by new social movements, both in the medical field and in the workplace. Finally, taking these struggles as an example, it will analyse how these movements brought about a new way of defining risk acceptance.

THE DEVELOPMENT OF A BIOLOGICAL APPROACH TO LEAD POISONING AS FROM THE 1960S

Until the early 1960s the most prevailing approach to lead poisoning in the workplace was the clinical one. Thanks to progress in international medical research, a biological approach based on urinary ALA (aminolevulinic acid) and coproporphyrins dosage allowing an earlier detection of lead poisoning has been developed. In 1972, in Amsterdam, an international conference dedicated to lead poisoning organized by both the CEC and the US EPA concluded that screening tests had to be based on biological indicators to detect the disease as early as possible.

In France, the progress of this medical knowledge had no positive impact on industrial lead poisoning screening for nearly twenty years. Even though after 1961 biological diagnosis of lead poisoning was the subject of French medical articles, until 1979 the French National Health Insurance continued to recognize only clinical parameters of lead poisoning thus compensating workers who were already poisoned. This reflected what several French social historians call 'the French culture of compensation' rather than prevention in the workplace when compared to other countries.

Even if early detection was medically possible at that time, this was not enough to change the criteria for lead poisoning recognition in the work place. During the 1970s, thanks to new social mobilizations, occupational health became an important issue for some physicians and rank-and-file workers.

NEW SOCIAL MOBILISATIONS FOR OCCUPATIONAL HEALTH

Mobilisations are reinforced in the wake of the 1968 social movement, which was challenging traditional authority in different areas of society. Medical students, practitioners and unskilled workers started protests related to occupational health issues.

During the 1968 events, medical power has been deeply criticised by students, general practitioners and some hospital doctors. They were pointing out the need to redefine the social role of medical practitioners and reduce the asymmetry of the doctor-patient relationship. At the time, these practitioners stated that "the medical field now belonged to everybody." This trend of thought gave birth to several groups. The major one was the French "Groupe Information Santé" (Health Information Group), founded in 1972. Even if numerically speaking, this Health Information Group was quite marginal, it had a real impact on medical practice concerning two social movements in the 1970s: the French women's movement for the right to abortion and the unskilled workers' strikes on health issues in the workplace.

During the 1970s, several strikes occurred in French factories. They were related to working conditions, especially those dealing with occupational health issues between 1972 and 1976. At that time, migrant workers went on strike in different factories with a main slogan: "Our health is not for sale." This was how they claimed prevention rather than a simple compensation for lead poisoning. Moreover, the struggle led by migrant workers in the Peñarroya factories shows that they wanted to be the ones to define risk acceptance criteria.

Definition of risk acceptance criteria

In the beginning of the 1970s in France, the two hundred Peñarroya migrant workers went on strike twice (1971-1972). They stood up for increased prevention in the workplace. According to the clinical diagnosis that was still dominant at that time, the Peñarroya company doctor did not recognize that they were poisoned by lead. The workers sought the help of medical practitioners from the Health Information Group to understand why they felt ill. Some politically committed practitioners agreed to help.

For several months in 1973, Peñarroya migrant workers and about ten general practitioners and medical students organized a cross-examination based on urine tests which concerned 27 of them. These tests were analysed by Professor Robert Zittoun, a famous hematologist in Paris together with the biologist Alfred Gajdos, one of the first French biologists who published a paper on lead poisoning subclinical diagnosis. According to biological features (the urinary ALA) 12 workers among the 27 were already poisoned by lead – presenting no clinical symptom.

These results had a double effect. Firstly, in February 1974, Professor Zittoun and Doctor Gajdos published an article in a French medical review – Le concours médical / Medical Assistance – dedicated to lead poisoning biological diagnosis. The Peñarroya Company reacted sharply to this article, and defended its policies by stating that this subclinical level of poisoning was an acceptable risk.

Henceforth, committed medical practitioners intensified mobilization. In 1975, they organised a national petition to claim for an earlier diagnosis of lead poisoning in the workplace. It was signed by hundreds of practitioners. At the same time, Peñarroya workers wrote a booklet entitled "How can workers get help from medical practitioners?" explaining this experience in their own words to other workers, and organized several meetings to distribute it in other lead factories all over the country. They also criticised the idea of this so-called risk acceptance threshold, explaining that it was up to them to decide what an acceptable risk was.

Moreover, in 1976, the French National Institute for Safety Research developed a urinary ALA easy to use test in the workplace. A year later, in 1977, the French Department for Labour and Social Security defined a new legal framework related to lead poisoning recognition in the workplace including urinary ALA biological diagnosis. After a seven-year long struggle, medical practitioners and migrant workers finally obtained what they claimed for: an earlier detection of lead poisoning in the workplace.

Conclusions

This case of social movement related to lead poisoning exposure in France shows the importance of medical knowledge progress but also proves that social factors are essential in such matters. Social factors have contributed to the definition of a new legislation on occupational disease recognition and prevention. The case also highlighted the role of the 'alternative' medical field in the development of occupational health issues at that time.

Challenging the "Blind Spots" of Expertise: Locally Produced Knowledge and Asbestos Hazard Management in Spain, 1975-1984

Alfredo Menéndez-Navarro
Department of History of Science
University of Granada, Granada, Spain

Social studies of science and the history of science have proven useful to challenge the expert explanatory model on the identification, management, and control of occupational risks.[1,2] Lay epidemiology and locally produced knowledge have been proposed as driving forces to inspire a more comprehensive approach to occupational hazards and to contest the traditionally social decontextualized views supported by experts.[3]

The aim of this paper was to explore alternative proposals to the expert model for the management and prevention of asbestos risks in Spain during the transition to democracy. While raw asbestos imports into Spain grew steadily from the early 1960s and peaked at 1974 (126,000 metric tons), the lack of commitment by Franco's Government and the low awareness of medical practitioners minimized public concerns about asbestos health hazards and the number of individuals awarded compensation. In 1974, only 40 asbestosis sufferers were officially entitled to compensation, and not a single case of cancer was recorded by the Ministry of Labor. In contrast, 40,205 silicosis sufferers were considered to be entitled to compensation.

By the mid-1970s, after the end of the dictatorship, the recovery of civil rights and the intensified mobilization of workers were crucial in stimulating public awareness on work-related health problems. The active stance taken by the Comisiones Obreras (one of the two most important general trades unions) in denouncing workplace carcinogenesis was in part inspired by the so-called Italian workers' model, developed in the late 1960s in industrialized Northern Italy. The model emphasized the value of locally produced knowledge, called for the direct intervention of workers in the assessment of risks and the control of working conditions, and sought to bring an end to the "monetarization" of risks and to the traditional delegation of these tasks to experts. The union's involvement was backed by young professionals, including medical researchers and union lawyers, who became increasingly engaged in asbestos occupational issues.

In 1977, concerns about asbestos entered the public sphere in Spain 1977. Non-compliance with safety and hygiene regulations by the Uralita fiber-cement factory in Cerdanyola (Barcelona) led the Barcelona Regional Board of Hygiene and Safety at Work to order the temporary closure of one wing of the factory. The conflict at Uralita forced the Government to take the bull by the horns. In May 1978, bronchial and lung carcinoma and pleural mesothelioma due to asbestos exposure were recognized as occupational diseases (RD 1995/1978, 12 May). In October of the same year, the Labor Department organized the First National Symposium on Asbestosis in Seville. The symposium agreed on a national plan for the health surveillance of exposed workers and on stricter technical regulations for the asbestos industry.

The alternative proposals made by Comisiones Obreras were mainly embodied in the report issued in 1982 by Francisco Báez Baquet (b. 1937), an office worker and member of the union at the Uralita fiber-cement factory in Seville. Báez Baquet's Report on asbestos and its hazards (1982), 4 which became crucial to the promulgation of national asbestos regulations in 1984, is a fine compilation of the expertise that he gained, drawing on both scientific evidence and contextualized local knowledge. Besides its value as a denunciation, the Report has three further strengths that derive from his use of a local contextualized approach to counter expert knowledge on asbestos risk. First, it reveals the author's awareness of the consensual nature of expert knowledge and how it can mediate medico-legal and preventive decision-taking. The identification by Báez Baquet of areas of medical uncertainty and his ability to draw on local knowledge to produce new evidence were crucial to his critique of expertise and to his call for workers to have a greater influence in the design and implementation of preventive safety measures. Second, the report highlights the reductionism of expertise and its decontextualized views on the management of occupational risks. Báez Baquet described flaws in the medical supervision of workers employed in scheduled areas, denouncing the exposure to dust of a greater number of workers than officially acknowledged. He called for regular medical examinations to be extended to ex-employees and also to workers' families and those living close to factories, challenging the radical separation between occupational and environmental sufferers. Concern was also expressed about the return to Spain of a growing number of emigrants, calling for special medical care and follow up for any who had previously worked in European asbestos factories. These and other proposals contrasted with the traditional neglect of social determinants of work in the expert approach to workplace risks, exposing what could be termed its 'blind spots'. Third, the report questioned the effectiveness of the technical control and safe handling of asbestos, raising concerns about the arbitrary nature of the threshold limits and their inadequacy, especially in relation to cancer risk. However, Báez Baquet accepted the need to be accommodating towards the unions on this issue, since unemployment rates were well over 16% in the early 1980s. At any rate, the Report called for the suppression of asbestos dust by technical means and for a reduction in exposure levels to be given priority over the "monetarization of risk."

The report backed the strong criticism by Comisiones Obreras of the first regulations, which were issued in 1982, and was also crucial in achieving an improvement in the National Asbestos Regulations issued in 1984 by the Socialist Government.

ACKNOWLEDGEMENTS

This research was supported by the Spanish Ministry of Science Project HAR2009-07543

REFERENCES

[1] Dembe AE. *Occupation and Disease: How Social Factors Affect the Conception of Work-Related Disorders*. New Haven: Yale University Press; 1996.

[2] Milles D. From Workers' Diseases to Occupational Diseases: The Impact

of Experts' Concepts on Workers' Attitudes. In: Weindling P, editor. *The Social History of Occupational Health*. London: Croom Helm; 1985. p. 55-77.
[3] Bloor M. The South Wales Miners Federation, Miners' Lung and the Instrumental Use of Expertise, 1900-1950. *Soc Stud Sci*. 2000;30:125-140.
[4] Báez Baquet F. Informe sobre el amianto y sus efectos nocivos. Sevilla: mimeograph; n.d. Historical Archive of Comisiones Obreras-Andalucía, Serie Francisco Báez Baquet, file 20.

The History and Impact of Presumptive Disability Laws for Firefighters

Taylor, JA[1], Phillips, JP[2], Hall, BL[3]
[1] Department of Environmental & Occupational Health, Drexel University School of Public Health, Philadelphia, PA, USA
[2] Department of History, Mississippi State University, Oktibbeha County, Mississippi, USA
[3] School of Law, Washington University in St. Louis, St. Louis, MO, USA

Background

The development of presumptive disability laws pertaining to occupationally-acquired diseases emanated from the application of the workers' compensation "injury by accident" prerequisite. Presumptive disability policy decisions react to the fact that unlike injuries, occupationally-acquired diseases are more difficult to prove as work-related. Due to the latency of diseases such as cancer, and the difficulty in establishing causation when disease manifestation may take decades, society made decisions to care for people whose occupations put their lives at risk. The creation of such policies began with the United States military, and subsequently expanded to first responders (police, firefighters). We present herein a concise history of presumptive disability law and an exploration of definitional and legislative issues that impact occupationally-acquired disease. Within this analysis, firefighters are used as a high-risk occupational group exemplar. We explore the prevalence, nature, and diversity of state-based firefighter presumptive disability laws within the United States and conclude by examining contemporary policy issues.

Materials and Methods

Historical Analysis of Federal Level Presumptive Disability Laws Applicable to the United States Military. We reviewed the twentieth-century evolution and development of federal level presumptive disability categories resulting from varied American war experiences. We placed particular emphasis upon such development within the context of geographic locale, tactical activities undertaken within the combat setting, and scientific advances specific to the study of disease pathology. Presumptive disability laws applicable within the military developed in the 1920s, commencing in 1921 with the establishment of presumptions for neuropsyciatric disease and tuberculosis and the dissemination of the first publication of chronic diseases to which presumptions would apply. These early presumptions found their genesis in the exposure of service personnel that in short temporal intervals resulted in disease but which were neither measured nor classified at the time of exposure Such early presumptive disability laws were grounded more on moral concern for returning veterans than scientific fact.

From the 1940s through the 1990s, federal Veterans Administration (VA) presumptions expanded as new exposures were experienced, and the science relating these exposures to disease were established. Congress and the VA have consistently expanded and clarified the scope of covered diseases, health outcomes, and disabilities within particular categories. This expansion and clarification has been particularly robust over the last twenty years. Presumption decisions increasingly rely upon statistical scientific evidence by which the presumption can be justified. However, legislation to include new categories of disease has not always arrived in time to help many of those affected. In 1991, legislation was passed to presume that all veterans who served in Vietnam between 1962 and 1975 were exposed to the defoliant Agent Orange. This sixteen year interval between the end of the war and the passage of legislation would have included average latency periods for many of the cancers the law eventually covered,[1] but because the law had not been developed, veterans may have manifested disease, been treated, and perhaps died before the benefit of the law could be realized. Categorically, health outcomes are currently structured under chronic diseases, tropical diseases, former prisoners of war, radiation, herbicide agents, mustard gas/lewisite, and Persian Gulf War.[2]

According to the International Association of Fire Fighters (IAFF), Pennsylvania created the first presumptive disability legislation for heart and lung disease in 1935.[3] Since then, approximately 40 states have followed, developing laws for a range of diseases for firefighters and other first responders. We present an analysis of these laws for the United States in the following section.

Analysis of Contemporary Status of State Level Presumptive Disability Laws Applicable to Firefighters

We reviewed public health literature, state statutes, and industry publications to evaluate the nature and extent of state level firefighter presumptive disability laws.[4] We principally relied upon a survey conducted by the International Association of Fire Chiefs. Within each disease type, we examined the extent and variety of coverage offered by individual states. We considered both the comprehensiveness and design of disease case inclusion criteria.

Results

Cancer

As a general proposition, cancer presumption laws stipulate that the state presumes cancers arising in firefighters result from carcinogenic exposures suffered during active firefighting duty. Seventeen states have enacted presumptive cancer laws that cover all forms of cancer in firefighters. In contrast, twelve states have passed legislation that covers a more limited universe of cancers. Twenty one states, along with the federal government, have yet to pass any form of presumptive cancer legislation.

Heart Disease

Twenty-nine states maintain laws covering heart disease that occurs among firefighters while five states cover acute myocardial infarctions suffered during and immediately following active firefighting duty. Heart disease legislation presupposes that occupational duties and stresses result in the increased risk of heart disease customarily observed in firefighters; accordingly, firefighters and their families receive access to compensation for incapacitating complications and deaths resulting from heart disease.

Infectious Disease

Eight states have presumptive laws for firefighters that cover all infectious diseases including for example HIV, hepatitis, meningitis, and tuberculosis; other states cover a limited number of infectious diseases, while most states cover none. Infectious disease laws presuppose, for the purpose of workers' compensation, that exposures suffered in the line of duty (including exposure to human blood) cause associated infections in firefighters. In most cases, proof of exposure and an absence of infection prior to such exposure constitute necessary conditions for receiving compensation.

Conclusions

Presumptive disability laws exist in most American states, and prove diverse with respect to disease inclusion and breadth. Inconsistencies in the laws may benefit from standardization. Adaptability needs to remain part of the design in order to accommodate unanticipated geographically-specific events such as the September 11, 2001 attack upon New York's World Trade Center. 5 Moreover, the changing face of firefighting has introduced new duties such as Emergency Medical Services (EMS) that present different hazards and outcomes, such as needlesticks and infectious disease. As with the evolution of laws for veterans, presumptive policies for firefighters need to change to reflect emerging hazards over time, and these adjustments need to be adopted broadly rather than by only a few states.

However, unlike the history of VA laws, presumptive legislation for firefighters should be promptly enacted following the emergence of new hazards.

Presumptive disability laws exist at the federal level for US veterans and at the state level for firefighters and other first responders. The federal government maintains its own fire service, for which no presumptive disability benefit exists. The Federal Firefighters Fairness Act approved by the Committee on Homeland Security and Governmental Affairs in 2009 awaits additional action.

References

[1] Weisenberger DD. Pathological classification of non-Hodgkin's lymphoma for epidemiological studies. *Cancer research* 1992;52(19 Supplement):5456s

[2] Samet JM, Bodurow CC. *Improving the presumptive disability decision-making process for veterans*. Natl Academy Press; 2008

[3] International Association of Firefighters. State Presumptive Disability Laws. International Association of Firefighters 2011 [cited 2011 Jan];Available from: URL: http://www.iaff.org/hs/phi/docs/PresumptiveDisabilityChart.pdf

[4] Williams N. HIV as an Occupational Disease: Expanding Traditional Workers' Compensation Coverage. *Vand L Rev* 2006; 59: 937

[5] Howard J. The World Trade Center Disaster: Health Effects and Compensation Mechanisms. *Journal of Law and Policy* 2007 Dec; 133 (69).

Abstracts as Presented

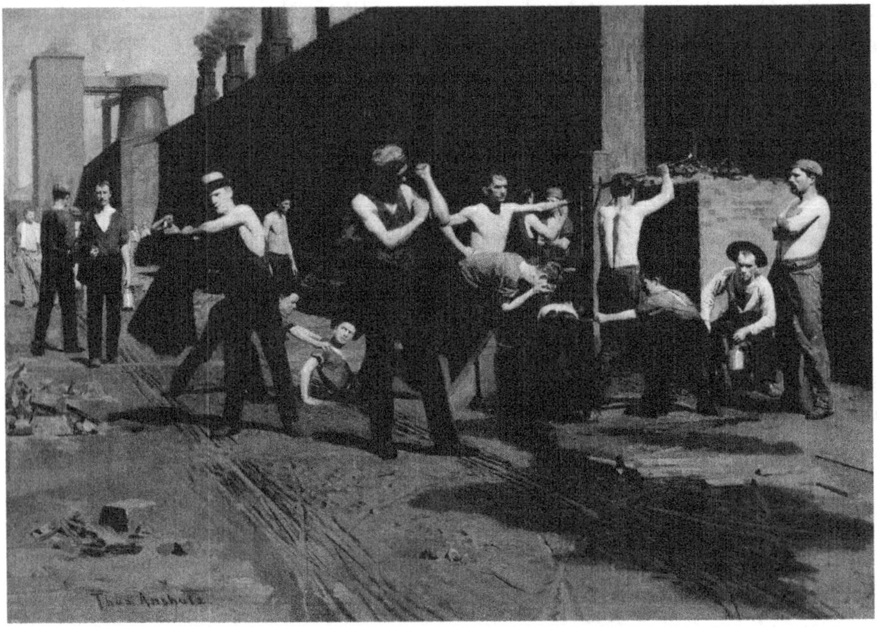

Ironworkers in factory yard: Thomas Pollock Anshutz, American, 1851¬1912 The Ironworkers' Noontime, 1880 Oil on canvas, 17 x 23 7/8 in. (43.2 x 60.6 cm).The Fine Arts Museums of San Francisco, gift of Mr. and Mrs. John D. Rockefeller 3rd, 1979.7.4.

The Life and Death of Gaius Julius Caesar From an Occupational Health Perspective

Jouni J.K. Jaakkola
Institute of Health Sciences, University of Oulu, Finland

The City of Rome was governed by kings until 510 BC, when the Lucius Iunius Brutus overthrew the king. During the republican era (509-27) the leading principle of governance was to prevent concentration of power. Annual appointment of two consuls was besides a safeguard against concentration of power, also a practice to reduce the influence of health problems to the leadership of the state. Fast expansion of Rome after the punic wars resulted insufficiency of the traditional form of government. After a civil war in January 44 Gaius Julius Caesar (100/2-44) was appointed as the first lifetime dictator (dictator perpetuus), which created a crisis of the republic. The experience of julio-claudian dynasty founded by Caesar's adopted son Gaius Julius Caesar Augustus (63 BC–14 AD) is an elaborate demonstration how problems of physical and mental health seriously influence the workability of an autocrat and the fate of the empire. The purpose of this study was to analyze the evidence of the illnesses of Caesar and their influence on his workability, i.e. capacity to lead the army and the state, and to consider how work may have influenced his health.

Contemporary writers (Cicero) and ancient historians (Appian, Cassius Dio, Plutarch, and Suetonius) who had access to extensive original documentary provide material on life events, habits and symptoms and signs of illness. Relevant ancient medical literature (Hippocrates, Celsus, and Galen) provides insight to contemporary concepts and practice of medicine. The analysis was based on original ancient texts describing Caesar's life and symptoms and signs of illness both from perspectives of ancient and modern medicine. Life course assessment was applied where health and illness are explained by hereditary factors, life habits, life events and work and family life.

There is evidence of a fever episode in 82 which may have been malaria. Direct descriptions of possible epilepsy attacks and complementary information support the hypothesis that Caesar suffered from epilepsy which may also have influenced his choice of life habits (restrictions of alcohol and diet) and action (fast decision making and action). Psychological and physical occupational strain may have worsened the epilepsy and there is evidence that Caesar was not able to lead the battle of Thapsus April 46 due to an epileptic attack; the experienced generals were able to win the day, but lost control of the after match which lead to a massacre. It seems possible that Caesar suffered two serious episodes of fatigue and depression which fit in the criteria of burnout syndrome; the first after Alexandrian War and the second in 45 in Rome. The latter episode manifestated in cynicism, depression, and lead to ignorance of safety measures which in the volatile political situation turned out to be fatal. He was murdered on 15 March 44. The succession of power required additional 15 years of devastating civil war.

The case study of Caesar indicates both the influence of work on health and health on work, and illustrates the vulnerability of autocracy to health problems of a dictator.

The Discovery of the Migrant Workers by Psychiatry

Benoit Majerus
Université libre de Bruxelles, Brussels, Belgium

In the 1960s and 1970s most European countries experienced a massive immigration of women and men from the Maghreb and Turkey, who often worked in low paid sectors. At the same psychiatry leaves the asylums and invested heavily on community care. Migrant workers is one of the new categories traditional psychiatry is confronted with in these years. In addition to practical problems, such as for example language barriers, the "selfwill" (Luedtke) of these patients often present a barrier to treatment. This 'new' patient requires different diagnoses, different treatment...

To illustrate this general European evolution, I will draw on a psychiatric hospital in Brussels. Using medical records from the 1960s and 1970s, I will compare the practice on a local level with national and international discourses (conferences, journals ...).

The concept of 'culture' serves as an umbrella term under which very heterogeneous differences that are often not tangible to the psychiatrist are tied together. Culture can be used here (1) to analyse interfamily relationships and conflicts (2) as an explanation for conflicts between countries of origin - and country of immigration and (3) to interpret misunderstandings between psychiatrists and patients. The years considered here are characterized by a large discrepancy between psychiatric discourse and practice. Only in the 1980s, occurs in the Belgian health care institutional solutions that fulfill the specific experience of partial migrants.

I am a researcher at the Department of History at the Université libre de Bruxelles. I'm working on a European history of psychiatry of the 20th century from below, a history based on patient records from three psychiatric hospitals (Berlin, Brussels and Paris).

Hospitality Workers' Exposure to Secondhand Smoke from 2006 to 2008 in Beijing, China

Ruiling Liu[1]*, Yanmin Lu[2], Yuan Jiang[3]

[1]School of public health, University of California at Berkeley, Berkeley, CA, USA; [2]Chinese Center for Disease Control and Prevention, Beijing, China. [3]Chinese Center for Disease Control and Prevention, Beijing, China.

Funding sources: This project was supported by a special grant from the Chinese CDC on FCTC annual implementation for 2007, and by a grant from the Roswell Park Trans-disciplinary Tobacco Use Research Center (P50 CA111236).

Background. In April 2004, China promised to hold a smoke-free Olympic Games in 2008 in Beijing; in January 2006, China became a party of WHO Framework Convention on Tobacco Control and is obligated to take effective measures to reduce SHS exposure. Mostly driven by these factors, China initiated a series of tobacco control activities in public places including hospitality venues. On Jan. 30, 2007, the Beijing Health Bureau and China CDC Tobacco Control Office called for hospitality venues to voluntarily prohibit or restrict smoking. On May 1st, 2008, the Beijing government implemented Regulations on Beijing's non-smoking Public Places, which includes a provision requiring restaurants to create separate no-smoking areas.

Objectives. The objective of this study is to investigate how has the hospitality workers' exposure to SHS changed with the social settings over three years from 2006 to 2008 in Beijing, China.

Methods. The study was conducted from 2006 to 2008 in Beijing, China, where hospitality venues were conveniently selected and both indoor and outdoor ambient air PM2.5 levels were measured using portable aerosol monitors. 92 venues were monitored from February to August in 2006, 85 venues from July to August in 2007 and 94 venues from October to December in 2008. 18 of these venues were followed up for all the three years.

Results. Among the monitored venues, 9.8% (9 of 92) completely prohibited smoking and 8.7% (8 of 92) restricted smoking to designated smoking area in 2006, these two proportions were 8.2% (7 of 85) and 2.4% (2 of 85) in 2007, and 55% (52 of 94) and 16% (15 of 94) in 2008. Among the 18 venues followed up for three years, only one venue prohibited smoking and one restricted smoking in 2006 and 2007, 6 venues prohibited smoking and 4 restricted smoking in 2008. In both 2006 and 2007, the median indoor PM2.5 level was lower than or similar to the median outdoor PM2.5 level for venues prohibiting or restricting smoking, while for other venues, the median indoor and outdoor level was 289 µg/m3 and 128 µg/m3, respectively, in 2006, and 248 µg/m3 and 126 µg/m3, respectively, in 2007. In 2008, the median indoor and outdoor level was about 75 µg/m3 and 53 µg/m3, respectively, for venues prohibiting or restricting smoking, and smoking was observed during sampling in 25% (13 of the 52) of the venues with complete bans. For venues without any smoking restrictions, the median indoor level was 81 µg/m3, comparing to the median outdoor level of 52 µg/m3. For the 18 venues, their median indoor PM2.5 level was 182 µg/m3 in 2006, 256 µg/m3 in 2007 and 93 µg/m3 in 2008, comparing to the median outdoor level of 82 µg/m3 in 2006, 123 µg/m3 in 2007 and 51 µg/m3 in 2008, respectively.

Conclusions. Hospitality workers' exposure to SHS during working was very high in Beijing, China in 2006 and 2007, and was reduced to some extent in 2008, but still not ignorable, which indicates that voluntary smoking policy does not work well, while governmental regulations and complete implementation seems necessary to protect workers from SHS exposure.

The Health of Sugarcane Workers in Brazil[1]

FLR Rocha, FLR,[1,2] MHP Marziale,[2] OS Hong, OS[3]
[1]*Supported by the Brazilian agency CAPES.*
[2]*School of Nursing of Ribeirão Preto of University of São Paulo. Ribeirão Preto, São Paulo, Brazil.*
[3]*School of Nursing of University of California, San Francisco, San Francisco, CA, USA.*

Background: Sugar cane was brought to Brazil after the Portuguese arrival, scattering with the help of the warm and humid tropical weather and the work force provided by African slaves. Initially, the cultivation of sugar cane prevailed in the Northeast of Brazil, expanding along the Brazilian coastline, mainly in the states of São Paulo and Rio de Janeiro. Nowadays, Brazil is the world largest producer of sugarcane. The state of São Paulo responds for around 65% of the national production, where 55% of the product turned into alcohol and 45% in sugar. The sugar cane agribusiness employs around one million Brazilian workers. About 40% of the sugar cane harvested is cut manually and the mechanization of sugar cane harvesting is rising significantly in the last years with the growing use of mechanical harvesters. During manual or mechanized cut, the workers are exposed to long daily shifts and to a workplace that presents several health-risk situations, such as high temperatures, rains, earth dust, soot from the burned sugar cane, venomous animals, occupational accidents caused by the handling of work instruments, accelerated rhythm of work and a set of repetitive corporal movements which favors the occurrence of accidents and musculoskeletal problems.

Materials and Methods: Field research with quantitative approach of the data, elaborated with the objective of analyzing the work and life situations that can offer risks to the workers' health involved in the manual and automated cut of the sugar cane. The sample was composed by 39 sugar cane cutters and 16 operators of harvesters. The data were collected during the months of July and August of 2006 by the technique of direct observation of work situations and workers' homes and through interviews, which were recorded and later transcribed. For the interpretation of the speeches, the technique of the content analysis was used. The research was structured according to the PRECEDE-PROCEED Health Promotion Planning Model. The presuppositions of the Social Ecological Theory, the Social Cognitive Theory and the Health Promotion Model were considered for the analysis of the data.

Results and conclusions: The workers' health is determined by the continuous interaction among several individual, environmental and social factors. Among these factors, it stands out the inadequate work and living conditions of the workers, who live in poverty. Concerning to work conditions, during the manual cut of the sugar cane the workers are exposed predominantly to the risk of occurrence of occupational accidents and the emergence of musculoskeletal diseases due to the adoption of incorrect postures, the execution of abrupt and repetitive movements and the intense corporal physical effort. In the automated cut, there is the predominance of risk of emergence of several psychological problems in the workers, arising from the constant demand of attention and concentration and in the ways of work organization, besides the risk of musculoskeletal problems due to the long permanence in the seating position. The data made possible the elaboration of a plan of interventions seeking the workers' health promotion.

Flame Retardants, Policy, and Public Health: Past and Present

Arlene D. Blum
University of California, Berkeley; Green Science Policy Institute, Berkeley, California, USA

In the 1970's, flammability regulations for children's pajamas, furniture, and baby products (strollers, baby carriers, high chairs, etc) were enacted to reduce fire deaths and injuries. These regulations were met by adding high levels of halogenated flame retardants to fabrics and polyurethane foam. Since then a series of toxic, bioaccumulative, and/or persistent organohalogen flame retardants have been removed from use due to their hazard to human health and the environment.

For example, in 1977, the Consumer Product Safety Commission (CPSC) banned brominated Tris [tris (2,3-dibromopropyl) phosphate] from children's sleepwear after it was found to be a mutagen, a carcinogen, and absorbed into children's bodies. The replacement, chlorinated Tris [tris (1,3-dichloro-2-propyl) phosphate], or TDCP, also a mutagen, was removed from use in pajamas, but not other products.

Beginning in the 1970s, the fire retardant pentabromodiphenyl ether (pentaBDE) was added to polyurethane foam in furniture and juvenile products to meet California's Technical Bulletin 117 (TB 117). PentaBDE is semi-volatile and migrates into dust. This organohalogen accumulates in humans, wildlife, and the environment and has the potential to cause adverse health effects. Legislation banning pentaBDE and also octaBDE was passed in California in 2003 and subsequently in eight other states and the EU.

The primary replacements in polyurethane foam are the same chlorinated Tris that was removed from children's sleepwear, and Firemaster 550, a mixture of four chemicals known to be toxic or lacking health information. In 2004, the EPA Design for the Environment predicted reproductive, neurological, & developmental toxicity and persistent degradation products from Firemaster 550, which is currently found in dust, sediment, and marine mammals.

In numerous animal experiments and a lesser number of human studies, pentaBDE and related fire-retardant chemicals have been reported to cause thyroid and endocrine disruption, reproductive, neurological, and developmental impairments, and cancer. Young children have about three times the levels of their mothers due to high levels in breast milk and dust. U.S. levels of PBDEs in house dust and body fluids are higher than those of other countries. Californian has higher levels than residents of other states. For the most highly exposed populations, the margin of safety for PBDE exposure appears to be low to non-existent for developmental neurotoxicity and reproductive toxicity.

However the California standard has not been shown to have reduced fire deaths in that state compared to other states which have no flammability regulations. The major causes of decreased U.S. fire deaths are less cigarette smoking, more smoke alarms and building sprinklers, childproof lighters, fire safe cigarettes and candles.

Recent attempts to alter California TB117 to reduce the use of halogenated flame retardants were defeated by chemical industry lobbyists. However, several industry proposals for requirements to increase the usage of unneeded flame retardants failed after peer-reviewed scientific research results were brought into regulatory processes.

Reducing halogenated flame retardants in consumer products appears to present an opportunity to contribute to preventing a wide range of adverse human health and environmental impacts without compromising fire safety.

Walt Whitman: An American Civil War Nurse who Witnessed the Advent of Modern American Medicine

DC Hsu

University of California, Davis Medical Center, Sacramento, CA, USA

Medicine in the 19th century underwent radical changes in its hospital organization, education, and sanitation protocols. Walt Whitman, at the age of 43, would serve as a voluntary Civil War nurse for seven years in the 40 hospitals of Washington, D.C. His poetry as recorded in the "Leaves of Grass" and "Drum-Taps" still serves as a testimony to that dreary state of pre-modern American medicine when expedient amputations were common, gangrene putrefied the air, and hygiene was woefully inadequate. It was a time when hospitals became divided into wards, which were managed by teams, and medical students received first-hand training. Whitman described how he dressed wounds and would stay up with soldiers into the night. In 1870, he ended his nursing career from a cut in his thumb that was slow to heal. This event prompted the beginning of the 20-year illness that would plague Whitman for the rest of his life. Although retrospective occupational hazards had surrounded his earlier nursing career, Whitman's later connections to American medicine as patient have provided historians a unique opportunity to explore the medical and psychiatric consequences of his role as nurse. Research shows that Civil War veterans are prone to a variety of physical and mental ailments.

The medical history of Walt Whitman as described by his doctors suggests that he may have suffered from psychosomatic illnesses, including post-traumatic stress disorder. Headache, congestion, malaise, insomnia, and constipation plagued Whitman on a daily basis. Although he eventually died of a pulmonary tubercular abscess, Whitman also suffered from three paralyzing strokes. Doctors by his side included the psychiatrist Dr. Richard Maurice Bucke, internist Dr. William Osler, and neurologist Dr. Weir Mitchell, as well as other physicians who cared for him to his death. Dr. Daniel Longaker performed Whitman's autopsy, including inspection of his brain. It was Longaker who stated that Whitman's illness originated from his hospital work, specifically "the emotional strain of those terrible years...[and the] blood-poisoning absorbed from certain gangrenous wounds in patients whom he at that time closely attended." Dr. Bucke, who was the founder of occupational therapy, was a close friend of Whitman, and would later write his first biography. By the time Whitman died in 1892, Osler had written his textbook on the practice of medicine, Lister had championed antisepsis, and Mitchell had described injuries of nerves.

Occupational health when Whitman served as a nurse was the product of larger social forces, specifically, the American Civil War. Similar to the Crimean War for European medicine one decade earlier, the American Civil War was the impetus for change in American medicine, and Walt Whitman remained in the center of it. Through the life and works of Whitman, historians can now appreciate the challenges that workers in the health professions faced just prior to the advent of modern American medicine.

The Magnificent Brown Family: Practitioners Caring for Workingwomen and Families, 1875-1925

Meredith Eliassen
San Francisco State University, San Francisco, CA, USA

In early 1875, Drs. Charlotte B. Brown and Martha E. Bucknell established the Pacific Dispensary Hospital for Women and Children as a public health model for indigent children and an urban clinical-training facility for female health professionals. Three and a half years after the Pacific Dispensary Hospital was founded, Kate Douglas Wiggin opened the Silver Street Free Kindergarten in the working-class Tar Flats neighborhood south of Market Street in San Francisco. Whereas the female medical practitioners inadvertently tread on male medical domain, Wiggin, who later becomes a best-selling author of children's books, utilized a perfect feminine vehicle for acclaim when she promoted the kindergarten movement in America. Houghton Mifflin and Company published Wiggin's The Story of Patsy, written to benefit the Silver Street Free Kindergarten in San Francisco, in 1889. In the book, Patsy with his "shrunken, somewhat deformed body," became a vehicle for promoting Wiggin's view of the spiritual potential of the kindergarten child in San Francisco's working-class communities, however the story also contained damning observations of working-class mothers.

While the Pacific Dispensary Hospital went about doing the gritty task of educating parents and the city about environmental and industrial health hazards, the kindergartner nurtured a romanticized worldview of ethereal child garden in San Francisco's slums. In 1896, Charlotte studied the health of adolescent schoolgirls 16 to 19 years of age in Oakland and San Francisco, to identify health problems appearing in immigrant and working-class communities that might be related to urban living. She found that the adolescent girls were suffering from similar health complaints to professional-women (teachers, typists, telegraph operators, and dressmakers), including dental, sinus, vision, and feelings of anxiety. Dr. Charlotte Blake Brown (1846-1904), and later her children Drs. Adelaide Brown (1867-1940) and Philip King Brown (1869-1940), became activists and proponents of preventative and occupational medicine for working families. The 1906 earthquake and fire brought about unique revelations for Charlotte's children. Adelaide, a gynecologist who managed the emergency room in the Presidio when hospitals were damaged, developed a career promoting the regulation of the milk industry to prevent bovine tuberculosis (the ailment afflicting Wiggin's character Patsy). Philip, a general practitioner with an interest in pulmonary medicine, compile in the wake of the 1906 earthquake and fire with its accompanying dust- and ash-filled air, statistics on the number of tuberculosis cases that were treated in his practice, and made the startling discover that the TB rate among working women was twice that of men. The reason for this was that women working in factories, shops, and as teachers were employed in closed quarters, in contrast to their male counterparts who often worked outside. The current treatment was bed rest, which was hard for women with familial responsibilities to achieve. This paper will look at how Drs. Charlotte, Adelaide and Philip Brown cultivated a new rhetoric in medicine to garner support for their mission of health equity and new forms of occupational therapy for women.

What is Worth Knowing, Experiencing and Sharing: Alice Hamilton and Contemporary Occupational Health Curricula

Leslie Anne Nickels
University of Illinois at Chicago School of Public Health, Chicago, IL, USA

Alice Hamilton (1869 -1970), considered a pioneer in industrial medicine in the United States, was an activist and physician who devoted her life to human rights and social justice and reducing workplace exposures and improving the health of workers. Her relentless pursuit in documenting workplace exposures in the early 20th century United States is the foundation of occupational health disciplines that today include industrial hygiene and occupational medicine. She distinguished herself through a career documenting what she believed was worth knowing and for using this knowledge to improve the lives of workers.

This paper will examine, through a curriculum inquiry of her life as a faculty member at Harvard, Alice Hamilton as an industrial medicine researcher and educator. Understanding how her work as an educator while at Harvard reflected what she thought was worth knowing, doing, and sharing in her commitment to healthy workplaces and ultimately her legacy in occupational health research and education. Her legacy includes; scores of research publications, legislation, and organizational awards given in her name, and is sustained through the contemporary occupational health disciplines of occupational medicine and industrial hygiene.

Research methods will include a comparative inventory of her work with the work of her United States contemporaries including government and peer reviewed publications and syllabi and course materials and an examination of her correspondence during her tenure at Harvard with her friends, family, colleagues and officials. I propose to understand 1) what she thought was worth knowing, experiencing and sharing; 2) how key aspects of Hamilton's education translated into the industrial medicine curriculum she pioneered at Harvard; and 3) ways in which her beliefs and methods are reflected in contemporary occupational medicine and industrial hygiene education.

In addition to gaining a better understanding of Alice Hamilton's contribution to occupational health in the 20th century, her relevancy is of is also of contemporary importance. The types of workplaces Hamilton investigated 100 years ago still exist today, to some extent in the US and extensively in many developing countries; workplaces with high levels of lead, silica, asbestos, and other contaminants, in places with dangerous workplaces and limited laws, enforcement and technical expertise to address the problems. In an effort to address the global burden of disease from workplace exposures, the World Health Organization is working on several fronts to increase awareness, build occupational health services capacity, and increase accountability of employers, activities that were Alice Hamilton's commitment to the workers in the US in 1909.

While Hamilton was an activist for human rights and social justice her success in bring attention and control to workplace hazards as a researcher and advocate during the nascent years of occupational health in the United States were universally acknowledged by industrialists, government officials, and academics. Understanding how she brought her experiences to the classroom can be understood through the lens of curriculum studies.

Helmut Valentin and the Institute of Occupational Medicine in Erlangen, Bavaria

J. Richard E. Thuerauf
Institute of Occupational Medicine, Erlangen, Germany

H. Valentin (1919–2008) and the Institute and Outpatient Clinic of Occupational, Social and Environmental Medicine, University of Erlangen-Nuremberg, are essential parts in the development of occupational medicine in the Federal Republic of Germany.

He had the first chair of occupational and social medicine in Germany, combined with an institute and a ward for the precise examination and care of patients suffering from occupational diseases. In the years from 1965 to 1989 the spectrum of tasks was permanently enlarged. His conception of a clinical orientated occupational medicine with integration of scientific analytical methods proved to be very successful.

His broad knowledge of internal medicine and experiences in cardiopulmonary function tests (developed by HW. Knipping, Cologne) favoured the start in Erlangen (where Friedrich A. von Zenker created the term "pneumoconiosis" (1867) and Franz Koelsch (1876-1970), first royal Bavarian "LandesGewerbeArzt" gave lectures). The intention was to explore the causes of health damages and to avoid them by using the best available methods and equipment. For example the body plethysmographs produced by Siemens, Erlangen, were used for lung function tests. The German Research Foundation (DFG) performed in 1965 – 1981 a multicenter epidemiological study on the significance of chronic inhalative burdens for the bronchopulmonary system. A total of 13,000 persons were examined, cross-section and follow up studies were combined to a longitudinal study to evaluate the effects of smoking habits, dust exposure and age. Due to his engagement in boards and committees Valentin could develop the official list of occupational diseases in Germany and the system of preventive medical examinations. Over 1000 scientific papers and several books were published.

Ambient monitoring was completed by Biological Monitoring (BM, dose and effect monitoring). Promoted by DFG, the Commission for the Investigation of Health Hazards of Chemical Compounds in the Work Area, Biological Tolerance Values for Occupational Exposure (BAT values) and Exposure Equivalents for Carcinogenetic Substances (EKA values) were established. The BM concept is now an element of the German legislation on health and safety at work. Numerous contributions came from the institute in Erlangen with its know-how – more than 100 parameters (metals, organic solvents, (non-)persistant pesticides, aromatic amines and nitro-compounds, polycondensated aromatic hydrocarbons, etc) and new possibilities arise from effect monitoring.

Valentin was dean of the Medical Faculty (1969-1970) and president of all German Medical Faculties (1971-1985), introduced occupational medicine as an obligatory discipline in medical education. As president of the German Society of Occupational Medicine and president of the Bavarian Academy of Occupational and Social Medicine, member of numerous expert boards and committees he was engaged on national and international levels to promote occupational medicine. Decorated with many honors he could as emeritus realize, that from his institute had developed the "Erlangen School" with eleven postdoctoral habilitations and representatives at the universities of Hamburg, Erlangen, Giessen, Berlin, Jena, Heidelberg, Mannheim, Freiburg, and even an academic "grandchild generation" in Aachen, Hannover, and Mainz: the enthusiasm for occupational medicine is still alive.

Working Conditions, Morbidity and Mortality at the Dutch Merchant Navy in the 17th and 18th Centuries: The Research of Arnold Leuftink

A.N. Weel

Centre of Excellence, Netherlands Society of Occupational Medicine, Utrecht, The Netherlands.

The Dutch occupational physician Arnold Leuftink [1918 – 1992] has made an impressive research into the historical sources of the Dutch mediconaval history. His thesis [1952] discusses the medical science in the Dutch Navy during the 17th century. After his retirement in 1982 he has spent all his time on the study of the working conditions, diseases and causes of death of seamen on merchant ships for the East. For this purpose he was staying a long period in foreign archives, especially in Cape Town, South Africa. Having processed all data he was able to describe a vivid picture of the hard life on board of the Dutch merchant ships of the United East Indian Company in the period of 1695 to 1795, especially during their travels from Holland to the Cape of Good Hope.

The most important primary sources for his research were the ship's journals and the so-called attestations from ship's surgeons.

In most ship's journals, a very accurate day to day bookkeeping of cases of death was found. In addition, extensive and often speculative descriptions of ship's doctors about the course of individual disease cases and their supposed causes were present. From our current knowledge of pathology it is possible to diagnose many of these cases.

From each travel a mortality diagram of the whole travel course was made. In studying these diagrams and combining their patterns with the other available data, Leuftink was able to assign certain diagnoses to specific patterns. Several specific epidemic patterns could be distinguished. This is the case for scurvy [scorbut], dysenteria, typhoid fever, typhus exanthematicus, yellow fever, bronchitis and pneumonia.

The results of Leuftink's research work (all publications are in Dutch language) are an important contribution to medical history. His approach of the sources and the way he has analysed the data are, although not perfect, an enrichment for medical historiography. Leuftink's approach and analysis will be presented at the Conference in San Francisco.

Italian workers' health between the two world wars of the 20th century

[1]Baldasseroni A, [1]Carnevale F, [2]Iavicoli S, [2]Petyx C, [3]Tomassini L.
[1]Local Health Unit of Florence, Florence, Italy. [2]ISPESL, Italian National Institute for Occupational Safety and Prevention, Rome, Italy. [3]University of Bologna, Bologna, Italy

Workers' health policy provides an important indicator to assess the whole range of social policies adopted during Fascism and to focus on the historical issue of continuity/discontinuity from Fascism to liberal state, widely discussed at national and international level.

The safeguard of workers' health became pivotal as the Fascist regime, after an initial liberal phase, launched a series of social policies that soon turned into the ideological scheme and identifying mark of Fascism.

After the murder of Matteotti and the enactment of the so-called "Fascistissime" laws and mainly after the promulgation of the "Carta del Lavoro" and the launch of the corporative state project, the world of work became one of the most relevant intervention fields of the Fascist domestic policies. In the early 30's, this attempt produced important results and led to the establishment of a highly centralized social insurance system divided into big institutions and able to act as a clearing house for the state-run financial bodies.

Health protection became one of the official and institutional instruments to get "consensus."

The Fascist policy on workers' health protection was deeply inspired by the ideology and general policy of the Fascist corporative state and based on the collaboration between capital and labour and the creation of the "authoritative modernization;" in addition, the strict workers' health and safety issues brought to light at least two clear contradictions.

The first one was about the industrialists. The corporate programme received tepid welcome or even a clear opposition from the representatives of the Italian industry that was experiencing typical marks of late comer countries. Employees wanted to have "idle hands" and exploited labour intensively, rarely abiding by the binding rules on the workers' health and safety prevention and protection.

In this regard, it is necessary to get documented answers to a series of questions, drawing upon official documents, special funds and a wealth of occupational health literature:

Did employees, who were entrusted the task of safeguarding workers' health, have the proper stimuli and rules to operate in this field?

Was the improvement of the public hygienic standards homogeneously planned and implemented also at workplaces? Or was it achieved in other health care sectors rather than workplaces?

Were the specific rules effective to monitor and reduce damage caused by the industrial and production expansion?

Finally, to what extent were the occupational health and physicians influenced by a culture and practices utterly subordinated to the power, more and more standoffish from the workers and laid down in a clinical and insurance niche irrelevant to the industrial hygiene and technical prevention?

The second clear contradiction lays in the gender issue and the so called "race defence," particularly relevant in the 30's. Long before Fascism turned into an overtly racist regime, health protection was pivotal in its family support strategies; in particular, women's health protection was strengthened because women, as mothers, safeguarded the pureness and the strength of the "Italic progeny." Nevertheless, the impetus towards eugenetics and demographic growth collided with the awful working conditions and the inadequate protection measure for female workers. These issues led to a series of institutional changes which redefined the state interventions in this area; however, the regime's ability to actually implement such new tools proved to be quite limited.

History of the Reporting of Occupational Disease in the Netherlands

Dick Spreeuwers

Netherlands Center for Occupational Diseases, Coronel Institute ; Academic Medical Center, University of Amsterdam, Amsterdam, Netherlands

Background: Most industrialized countries have one or more registries of occupational diseases. These national registries are often linked to a financial compensation system for occupational diseases that is embedded in the country's social security system. The pattern of occupational diseases has been changed in the last century from "classical occupational diseases", like silicosis and lead poisoning, to "modern occupational diseases" like musculoskeletal disorders and mental health problems. Since 1911 five different reporting systems for occupational diseases have been used in the Netherlands, based on different legislation and with various goals, reporters and results.

Materials and methods: We performed a literature search to compare five different reporting systems for occupational diseases, which have been used in various periods in the Netherlands since 1911. We surveyed which legislation the registration was based on, the official goals of the registration, the persons responsible for reporting and the results of the registration. On the basis of these elements we tried to explain the trends in statistics of occupational diseases in the Netherlands.

Results: From 1911 all physicians in the Netherlands were obliged to report occupational diseases to the Labour Inspectorate. The scheme was set up for preventive purposes and was not linked to compensation. Physicians received a small reimbursement for every notification. The scheme did not yield many notifications: maximum 500/year. This scheme was finally abolished in 1971.

Since 1928 a few defined occupational diseases had to be reported to the National Security Bank for compensation purposes. Insurance physicians were responsible for the recognition of the notifications. This scheme finished with the introduction of the Work Disability Act in 1967, which did not make a distinction between diseases caused by work or by other sources.

Since 1967 insurance physicians had the obligation to report occupational diseases. In fact the assessment of an occupational disease was irrelevant for the assignment of a disability pension, which resulted in a lack of interest in registration of occupational diseases in the Netherlands. As a result there was hardly any information on occupational diseases in the Netherlands in the eighties. A new scheme for reporting started in 1989. All employers were obliged to report occupational diseases tot the Labour Inspectorate. This scheme had some success: the number of reports increased during the nineties.

Since 1999 Occupational Health Services are legally obliged to report occupational diseases to the Netherlands Center for Occupational Diseases.

The number of notifications is about 6000 per year since then.

Conclusions: In all schemes there is a considerable level of underreporting and selective reporting.The large number of musculoskeletal disorders is not a recent trend in the Netherlands. Already in the sixties 25% of the reported occupational diseases were musculoskeletal disorders. In older schemes occupational skin diseases were on top of the list of reported occupational diseases, whereas only 2-3% of the current notifications are skin diseases. The explanation is that reporting today is closely related to sickness absence guidance and employees with skin diseases tend to continue working.

Development Process of Occupational Health Nurses in South Korea

Kyung Ja June,[1] G Yi,[2] YM Kim,[3] SY Kim,[4] O Hong[5]
[1]Dept. of Nursing, Soonchunhyang University, Chonan-si, South Korea
[2]Dept. of Nursing, Sangi University, Wonju-si South Korea
[3]Busan Combined Cycle Power Site Division, Busan, South Korea
[4]Korea Occupational Safety and Health Agency, Incheon, South Korea
[5]Department of Community Health Systems School of Nursing, UCSF, San Francisco, CA, USA

The purpose of this study is to describe the development process of occupational health nursing and to analyze the influence of social, political, and professional factors on the development. Secondary analysis and case study were done for this purpose. In Korea, occupational health nursing has been developed in four stages. The first stage is the period before 1980 when nurses had been working in industries as the first aid personnel without any specific legal base. Since 1981, nurses have been recognized as occupational health professionals. However, the role of the occupational health nurse was limited to providing direct service at the plant dispensary. After the amendment of Occupational Safety and Health Law in 1991, the role of occupational health nurse was expanded as an occupational health manager who performs the responsibilities similar to physicians or industrial hygienist. As the result of job delineation study, occupational health nurses recognized more importantly the role of occupational health nurse as direct care provider than educator, consultant or manager. In 2003, occupational nurse specialist certification system was established with other advance practical nurse certification system by Medical Law. One master program for occupational health specialist has been opened, and Korean Accreditation Board of Nursing conducted the first qualification examination in 2006. From this development process, influencing factors including social, political, and professional aspects will be discussed to suggest the future direction.

Medical History for Aircraft Maintainers: A Look to the Future

James W. Allen
Working Healthy Always, LLC

Background

When World War I started powered flight was only ten years old. Aircraft were made of fabric and wood with construction techniques that involved painting a solution onto linen fabric. Early in the war aircraft factories at both England and Germany experienced the death of maintainers constructing aeroplanes. Research in occupational exposures revealed the cause. In the 1930s aircraft construction changed from wood and fabric to aluminum. This change permitted more rapid construction of complex shapes required for the advances in aeronautics. The large workforces used in WWII experienced new exposures associated with metal construction. Currently a dramatic shift is occurring in aircraft construction. Aluminum is giving way to composites which are now present in modern airlines, military aircraft, and rotor and turbofan blades. A view of exposures from past aircraft construction techniques will alert aircraft maintainers about potentially unseen exposures resulting from the new composite construction.

Material & Methods

Review of medical literature from WWI and WWII contains studies about construction techniques that placed maintainers at risk from their work on aircraft. One report from WWI reflects a public health warning by Alice Hamilton and the ones from WWII anticipate future exposures. Review of these medical reports leads to trade publications that address exposures from aircraft construction. Current aviation trade journals highlight the ongoing shift to composite construction techniques.

Results

Wood and fabric aircraft required the linen be taught and fireproof. Doping was the technique used to apply a chemical solution that contained Tetrachloroethane. This chemical meets the engineering requirements, offered a sweat fragrance to the workers and was thought to be non toxic. This latter misconception followed the current logic that the skin was impenetrable and carbon tetrachloride was the most toxic chlorinated hydrocarbon. Both assumptions were wrong as the death of aeroplane workers in England and Germany documented. Aluminum construction in WWII used power tools for shaping and coatings for subsequent painting. A study at the Douglas Aircraft factory showed aluminum and its coatings as the cause of contact dermatitis. Similar exposures also caused contact dermatitis at the Aerospatiale factory from 1981 to 1990. A study of vibrating tools at another aircraft facility documented the frequency and risk factors for hand arm vibration syndrome. Forty year later a NIOSH study at the Gulfstream Aerospace Corporation documented defective powered tools that could cause similar effects. As aircraft construction moves to composites, maintainers come in contact with adhesives and fiber reinforced laminates. Plastic composite workers from Finland experienced more dermatitis. Other medical reports include nerve damage from N-hexane exposure, testicular cancer from dimethyformamide and mood disorders from solvent exposures.

Conclusions

Dramatic shifts in primary construction material for aircraft have occurred in the past. When previous transitions occurred to wood and fabric and then metal aircraft, maintainers experienced unanticipated health effects. The current transition to composites suggests that unanticipated medical effects will occur among aviation maintainers.

The History of Airline Medicine in the United States

Robert R. Orford

Mayo Medical School and Consultant, Division of Preventive, Occupational and Aerospace Medicine, Rochester, MN, USA

Commercial aviation began in the United States in the 1920s, and almost from the beginning, physicians were employed to medically evaluate new employees, and to provide occupational medical services for air crew and ground crew. Early airline medical directors included Dr. Ralph Green of Eastern Airlines, Dr. Edward Greene of American Airlines, Dr. Arnold Tuttle of United Airlines, Dr. Jan Tillisch of Northwest Airlines, and Dr. Kenneth

Dowd of Tran Canadian Airlines. As the industry grew, the complexity of the role of the Airline Medical Director evolved, to include the assessment and management of human factors such as ergonomics of cockpit and cabin design, circadian rhythm disturbance resulting from long haul flights, and cosmic radiation. The Airlines Medical Directors Association was founded in 1944, not long after the origin of commercial aviation in the United States, and has annually brought together medical directors and present and former medical department staff from airlines in the US and around the world. The Medical Committee of the Air Transport brings together active medical directors of US and Canadian airlines several times each year to discuss topics of current interest such as the Air Carrier Access Act, the passenger medical kit, the use of defibrillators on aircraft, and pandemic influenza. The speaker will review the history of airline medicine in the United States from his perspective as former Joint Medical Director of Northwest Airlines, and as a member of both the Airlines Medical Association and the Medical Committee of the Air Transport Association.

History of Construction Safety and Health

Knut Ringen

CPWR: The Center for Construction Research and Training

The construction industry is one of the largest economic sectors, and also one of the most hazardous, with fatality and injury rates that typically are three times greater than its contribution to employment. Nevertheless, the industry has received relatively little attention in the occupational safety and health community, and the history of occupational safety and health in this industry has never been explored systematically. To begin to remedy this void the ICOH Scientific Committee on Occupational Safety and in the Construction Industry is beginning to collect and systematize the historical evidence. This presentation is the first output from this effort.

The history covers the last 130 years and falls in two distinct categories, and we will present evidence from both of these:

- Safety can be traced to responses to large disasters, such as bridge collapses, explosions, etc. Some of these are well known such as the Golden Gate bridge and Gauley Bridge Tunnel, but there are many other significant events internationally that have received little attention.
- Health can be traced to the emergence of construction industry wel-

fare organizations in Europe, beginning in Germany with Bismarck's reforms, and generally parallels the history of social medicine.

In addition, we will give an overview of the emergence of a scientific basis for construction safety and health over the past 40 years, in which the Scientific Committee has had a significant part. We hope the outcome of this presentation will be to stimulate more interest in the history of construction safety and health, and that other participants will share evidence they have uncovered that may be relevant to this undertaking.

Prevention of Occupational Noise-Induced Hearing Loss: Past, Present, and Future

Madeline J Kerr, OS Hong, & RT Sataloff
University of Minnesota, Minneapolis, MN; University of California, San Francisco, CA; Drexel University, Philadelphia, PA, USA

Promoting hearing health is a national priority in the United States. Recognizing the universal risk of noise exposure, the Healthy People 2020 initiative is retaining two objectives to prevent hearing loss in the noise-exposed public: 1) increasing use of ear protective devices and 2) reducing the proportion of adults who have elevated hearing thresholds or audiometric notches, in high frequencies (http://www.healthypeople.gov/hp2020). Recent epidemiological studies by the National Institute for Occupational Safety and Health (NIOSH) indicate that work-related hearing loss continues to be a serious health and safety issue in the United States. Using data from the National Health and Nutrition Examination Survey, NIOSH estimated that more than 22 million workers in the United States were exposed to hazardous noise, and that one in four workers did not use hearing protection devices.

In this presentation, approaches to occupational noise-induced hearing loss prevention in the United States over the past half century will be described using a hierarchy of controls framework and a multidisciplinary perspective. Historical data will be mined from books, such as the textbook by Joseph Sataloff (1957), and archival records such as the historical timelines of the Occupational Safety and Health Administration, NIOSH, the Council for Accreditation in Occupational Hearing Conservation, and the National Hearing Conservation Association. Contemporary research publications will be cited to represent the state of the science in occupational noise-induced hearing loss prevention. The ideals of engineering controls to eliminate hazardous noise, and administrative controls to remove workers from the hazard, have yet to be realized in workplaces across the nation. Therefore, our emphasis will be on the third element in the hierarchy of controls, hearing protection for every noise-exposed worker.

We will trace the evolution of hearing protection education and training methods, from one-on-one and group classroom instruction, to video plus hands-on practice with a classroom instructor, to the more recent free-standing computer-based education with independent hands-on practice. We will explore future educational methods to reach the widespread global workforce through mobile technology. Finally, we will address prevention program evaluation methods with a vision towards standardized electronic record-keeping and a future of interoperable electronic health records for every worker. Aggregating workers audiometric data and their hearing protection education records will enable organizations to evaluate hearing loss prevention programs internally. Organizations will also be able to benchmark their performance in comparison with national reference statistics as NIOSH establishes their new surveillance program for occupational noise-induced hearing loss. As history reveals, together the many disciplines involved in hearing loss prevention can make a difference for noise-exposed workers.

Surviving the "Long Turn:" Overwork and Sleep Deprivation in the Early-Twentieth-Century American Steel Industry

Alana V. Derickson

Pennsylvania State University, University Park, PA, USA

The effects of overwork and sleep deprivation, especially related to non-standard work schedules, are now understood to include shift-work sleep disorder, gastro-intestinal ulcers, and other acute and chronic diseases. A century ago, when sleep medicine and sleep science did not exist as established fields of inquiry, these effects were less well recognized. Nonetheless, the turn of the twentieth century witnessed a dawning awareness of the adverse consequences of disrupted and diminished rest for workers.

This paper explores working time as a significant hazard for workers in the burgeoning and rapidly evolving American steel industry. Continuous operations in steelmaking entailed unconventional hours on duty. The imbalance of power between employers and employees led to extremely long hours at work and biorhythmically unnatural rotational arrangements. During the industrializing era, a substantial share of US steel workers toiled for twelve hours a day, seven days a week, and rotated between days and nights every two weeks by completing a twenty-four-hour stint known as the "long turn." In the absence of scientific investigation of this onerous regime, lay observers did provide many insightful observations of the deleterious impact of chronic sleep deprivation for employees. These analyses illuminated not only strenuous toil and inadequate sleep but also the crowded, noisy places in which workers had to try to rest after work. Widespread and growing dissatisfaction with this unhealthful system led in 1919 to the largest strike in American history up to that time. Although the strike failed, public scrutiny of this set of employment relations and other factors soon thereafter brought about the end of the twelve-hour day and the "long turn."

This paper rests on research in the records of the Interchurch World Movement (mediators of the 1919 labor dispute) and other manuscript sources. It also draws on numerous published contemporary accounts of working conditions produced by journalists, Progressive reformers, unionists, industry representatives, government officials, and workers themselves.

One to Five: The Remarkable Moment in Intellectual History that Created the ILO Encyclopaedia

Ilise L Feitshans
University of Lausanne, Lausanne, Switzerland

"To love one's work is a blessing, but where is the work that loves us?" (Albert Thomsa, First Director of ILO in the Preface to the first edition.)

The International Labour Office (ILO) is the oldest specialized agency of the United Nations, founded in 1919 under the Treaty of Versailles. The ILO Encyclopaedia of Occupational Health and Safety is an internationally respected standard reference. Accuracy, objectivity and commitment to its international mission have been the hallmark of the Encyclopaedia since 1930. Albert Thomas wrote: "In 1919 the International Labour Conference at Washington rccjue.sted the International Labour Office '' to draw up a list of the principal processes to be considered as unhealthy. But it was impossible in practice to draw up such a list. These considerations led to the idea of substituting for the list of unhealthy processes requested by the Conference, a sort of ency'ctopoedia which would analy'se from the triple point of view of the work to be done, the worker employed, and the environment in which he worked, the various tasks involved in human labour, the properties of the substances dealt with, the operations involved in handling and 'working up these substances, the possible sources and carriers of intoxication and disease, the statistical data on the effects as far as known, the symptoms, the diagnosis, the therapeutic and prophylactic treatment, and the protective legislation already in. existence... They must, however, have already found the first and greatest recompense for their work in the work itself. Each of them is an apostle as well as an expert in his own country. ... The Preamble to Part XIII of the Peace Treaty included among the urgent tasks of the Office the protection of workers " against sickness, disease and injury arising out of their employment ". The signatory States, in agreeing to this statement of principle, seem to have accepted the dictum of Lord Beaconsfield, that the health of the people is the most important of all problems. The Office is proud to think that it may perhaps claim the merit of having provided for the first time since the war the means and habit of intellectual co-operation, irrespective of frontiers, for the welfare of all ."

Therefore the first edition of the ILO Encyclopaedia of Occupational Health and Safety was a remarkable moment for intellectual history. When Dr Alice Hamilton and her colleagues wrote for the First Edition they invented what we call the "right to know". Using materials from the ILO archives, this paper explores how they did this important work.

Creating Environmental and Occupational Health in the Twentieth Century: A Journal, its Editorial Board, and the Field it Shaped

DR Smith[1] and TL Guidotti[2]

[1] *University of Newcastle, Ourimbah, New South Wales, Australia*

[2] *Washington, DC, USA*

Although the historical development of environmental and occupational health (EOH) in the United States (US) has been well-recorded in the academic periodicals of this field, journals that were prominent in the past, especially before 1980, may not be well-known by contemporary practitioners, while name changes may have further obscured the continuity of publication. One of the longest running and most influential EOH journals in this regard is the Archives of Environmental & Occupational Health (AEOH), a periodical which can trace its roots back to 1919 when originally founded as the

Journal of Industrial Hygiene (JIH) by the then-Dean of Harvard Medical School, David Edsell. Published by the then newly-formed Industrial Medical Association, now the American College of Occupational and Environmental Medicine, the JIH can lay claim to being one of the first English-language periodicals dedicated solely to EOH.

Through a series of name changes, affiliations and publishers during the 20th century, the journals' editorial boards featured a selection of prominent leaders in EOH, including Edsall and the Drinker brothers, as well as several pioneering women in the field, such as Alice Hamilton and Katharine Boucot Sturgis. The journal also served a pioneering role in the collection and dissemination of scientific data throughout last century, publishing many articles that would later become EOH classics, including some that would serve as the foundation for statutory regulations in the US. By the 1970s the journal, then publishing as the Archives of Environmental Health (AEH), had become a significant source for US air quality standards. During early years of the new US Environmental Protection Agency for example, a watershed era for US environmental protection standards, the AEH served as a major outlet for crucial air pollution research such as the Community Health and Environmental Surveillance Studies (CHESS).

In the twentieth century the AEOH continues to provide valuable source material for significant historical research on occupational and environmental health. For nine decades between 1919 and 2009, through numerous publishers and editorial boards, seven different titles, and two World Wars, the AEOH in its various incarnations has disseminated findings to an ever-changing audience. Equally importantly, it has served as an instrument to shape the agenda for occupational and later environmental health research at several key periods in the evolution of the field. This historical review demonstrates the roles of EOH journals beyond archiving scientific information, including the cultivation of a new scientific endeavor, serving as a forum for debate in emerging fields, establishing an agenda for significant problems in the field, and encouraging new scholars.

Conflict of Interest Declaration

The authors, Derek R. Smith and Tee L. Guidotti, currently serve as Deputy Editor-in-Chief and Editor-in-Chief respectively, of the Archives of Environmental & Occupational Health.

Preliminary Explorations in the ACOEM Archives

Tee L. Guidotti
Past President, American College of Occupational and Environmental Medicine; Washington DC, USA

The archives of the American College of Occupational and Environmental Medicine (ACOEM) are a valuable source of information on the history of occupational medicine in the United States. The archives constitute paper files of approximately 25 linear feet. They include complete verbatim transcriptions, typed on onionskin paper, of board meetings until the 1960s, when an "action item" format was adopted for minutes. These documents are now fragile. Accurate interpretation of the records requires knowledge of the individuals, their positions at the time, and the context.

In the summer of 2007, I examined the ACOEM archives to determine the scope of their contents. Because of time limitations I concentrated on the decadal years from 1940 to 1990 and on the early 1950's, when occupational medicine, represented by the then-named Industrial Medical Association, together with the movement for national health insurance and prepaid medical services was in a three-sided conflict with the American Medical Association and the American Public Health Association. In 1952, Carey McCord (a prominent occupational physician and toxicologist) vetted a speech he proposed to give to the AMA Section on Public Health and Preventive Medicine with the Board of Directors of the Industrial Medicine Association (IMA), as ACOEM was then known. He took issue with an article published by Herbert Abrams (a famous advocate of public health and national health insurance who later became head of the occupational health program at the University of Arizona) advocating integration of occupational health services with public health services at the local level and absorption of occupational health into public health. McCord said specifically toward the end of his remarks that he had no quarrel with public health. However he thought that occupational medicine was a distinct specialty so technically complicated that it should stand alone. This suggests that the divisions between the APHA and IMA were based on professional and technical differences, not ideology.

On the other hand, in the 1940s and 1950s, there was a strong feeling of alienation toward the AMA, which was opposing all forms of organized health care, including employer-sponsored healthcare for workers, and had established an unrepresentative Council on Industrial Health that competed with and often contradicted the IMA by siding with general practitioners opposed to changes in healthcare. At the same time IMA leaders were ambivalent because felt they that the AMA occupational medicine had nowhere else to go to get its views heard. The deep and bitter division between the AMA and the IMA is not generally known.

Further exploration of this valuable resource will depend on rendering the files into a searchable electronic format. A fuller picture of the evolution of the field would be obtained by comparing the ACOEM record of deliberations on the same issues with that of the AMA and APHA.

The Wieliczka Salt Mine: An Account of how Improved Workers Health Jumpstarted the Field of Speleotherapy

AL Redford, ML Zaremba, KM Elliott, SP Reddy
St. Clair Pulmonary & Critical Care, Port Huron, Michigan, USA

Background

Working conditions have been known for a long time to contribute to the burden of disease. Creation of unique and novel disease states and subsequently innovative measures to control disease incidence and prevalence have been fashioned. We attempt to show somewhat of the opposite where we believe a healthy work environment for workers with respiratory diseases may have contributed to novel treatment and rehabilitation of patients with respiratory disease and help conceptualize a new mode of treatment Speleotherapy.

Material and Methods

Wieliczka, a small town in Poland, had once been the economic hub of Poland due to the discovery and commercialization of Salt. This resulted in a network of elaborate tunnels rooms and halls.

In the 19th century a young physician named Feliks Boczkowski was inspired by balneology, a treatment using brine baths, which was quite fashionable and used to treat many ailments. He also noticed that the miners did not suffer from lung disease and set up a spa based on these findings. Before these spas could be brought to their great magnitude a cholera epidemic erupted and closed them down with its founder dying while caring for these patients. Later, approximately 100 years in 1958, Professor Mieczyslaw Skulimowski noticed the beneficial effects of this unique environment on the health of workers with lung disease. This resulted in the attempt to setup a Rehabilitation environment for patients with lung disease.

The history of the creation of one of the oldest salt rehabilitation centers for patients with asthma is explored by the examining of the mine itself, documents and accounts from a variety of sources.

RESULTS

Beneficial experiences of workers with lung disease seem to have led to the formal creation of a novel form of therapy, Speleotherapy.

CONCLUSION

Unique work environments may cause unique disease states but are also an opportunity to observe the natural history of disease resulting in newer forms of treatment as evidenced by the Wieliczka experience. Due to the lack of economic benefit in mining salt, in abandoned salt mines, these mines may be harnessed to improve the health of severe asthmatics thanks to observations on hard working people with respiratory disease.

Courting Clio: Historians and their Testimony in Products Liability Litigation

NA Schachtman* and JA Ulizio[1]

Lawyer in private practice.

[1]*Lawyer, and Chief Executive Officer of U.S. Silica Co., New York, NY, USA*

Parallel developments in mid-20th century medicine and American tort law resulted in the need to resolve factual disputes about events several decades old. After World War II, epidemiology developed the assessment of case-control and cohort studies to permit reliable detection and quantification of causal associations between diet, medications, social habits, and occupational or environmental exposures and various chronic diseases. Latency periods, often decades long, complicated but did not prevent the identification of causes of cancer and other diseases – such as tobacco, asbestos, DES, radiation, among others.

Also in the middle of the last century, American law evolved to extend manufacturers' and sellers' duties in tort to prevent harm from defective products, not only to immediate purchasers but to all foreseeable users. Contributory fault, which had barred recovery, gave way to comparative fault, which only reduced damages. Most important, statutes of limitations, which previously barred suits filed after two years or so from last exposure, were modified to permit suits within two years of when the claimant's injury became clinically manifest and discoverable. With these developments, injured workers became entitled to sue for injuries caused by products, even though the causal exposures occurred decades earlier.

These advances in epidemiology and tort law have put into issue factual disputes over who knew what about product risks, many years before the injury and the lawsuit. Parties on both sides have struggled to interpret old medical texts and documentary evidence, on evidentiary records often incomplete and ambiguous. The meaning of the old scientific evidence was typically beyond the ken of ordinary laypersons, and thus litigants sought expert witnesses, with expertise in historical methods or medical science, or both, to explain and present the historical evidence.

The advent of historian expert witnesses in tort cases has raised legal questions about how courts should supervise and control the reliability and advocacy of historian witnesses. The narrative typically created by historians threatens to usurp the lawyers' role in interpreting and arguing the evidence and inferences to the jury, and the jurors' role in finding the facts from the evidence in the case.

The early judicial response frequently relied upon vigorous cross-examination to reveal historians' use of incomplete or misleading evidence. More recently, legal writers have criticized judicial passivity in the face of tendentious historical expert opinion testimony. Various proposals, ranging from heightened judicial scrutiny and gatekeeping for historian witnesses, to appointment of neutral witnesses, to eliminating or reducing the scope of historians' testimony, have been suggested. Recent case law shows no clear path to resolving the difficulties inherent in the reliance upon historians' opinion testimony in tort cases.

The history of the occupational disease silicosis, and historians' testimony in the litigation of silicosis claims over the last two decades, will be used as a case study of the utility and dangers in having historians serve as expert witnesses.

Epilogue

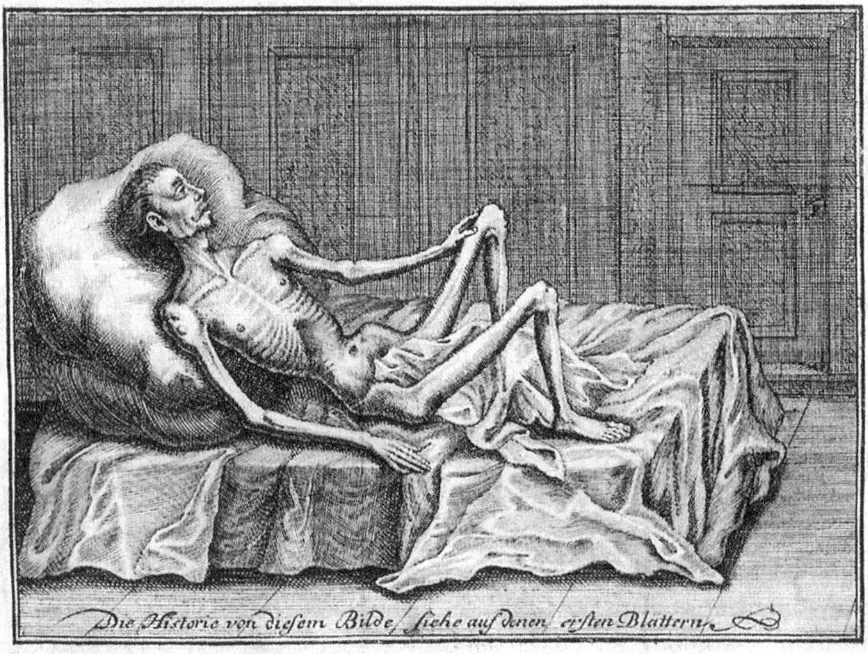

"Tod an Bleyvergiftung." Illustrated in: Georg August Ebell, Die Bleyglasur des irdenen Küchengeschirrs als eine unerkannte Hauptquelle vieler unserer Krankheiten und Mitursache der Abnahme körperlicher Kräfte der Menschen, besonders der höheren Stände : aus gerichtlichen Verhören und andern Beweismitteln dargethan (Hannover: [Selbstverl.], 1794). Original 15 cm by 9 cm. A similar copper plate image appeared in an earlier publication: Johann Friedrich Henckels, Aufstand u. Schmelz-Bogen von d. Bergsucht u. Hütten-Katze, auch einigen andern, denen Bergleuten u. Hütten-Arbeitern zustoßenden Krankheiten, vor dieselben u. diejenigen, so in Stein, Erz, Metall u. Feuer arbeiten ausgestellet (Dresden; Leipzig: Joh. Friedrich Henkels [Henckels], 1745).

Speaking about the Other:
On the Relevance of the Humanities to Occupational Health

Brian Dolan, PhD
Professor of Social Medicine and Medical Humanities
University of California, San Francisco, San Francisco, CA, UA

In the late 1930s, the British mathematician Godfrey Hardy posed a question to his friend C.P. Snow. "Have you noticed how the word 'intellectual' is used nowadays?" he asked. "There seems to be a new definition which certainly doesn't include Rutherford or Eddington or Dirac or Adrian or me. It does seem rather odd, don't y' know."[1]

Hardy was soon to publish a book called *A Mathematician's Apology* (1940) on the aesthetics of mathematical thought written for a lay audience, the forward to which was written by Snow. Also in 1940, Snow, a Cambridge don and physical chemist, would publish his first of a series of political novels that would make him a minor celebrity amongst the British literati. However, what Hardy had said to him provoked reflections on contemporary society that Snow later articulated in a public lecture at Cambridge in 1959 and which was published under a title that would make him far more famous: "The Two Cultures and the Scientific Revolution."

Both Hardy and Snow were scientists who sought to communicate both technical and creative ideas to a wide public. Hardy, to be sure, had written that "the mathematician's pattern's, like those of the painter's or the poet's, must be beautiful, the ideas, like the colours or the words, must fit together in a harmonious way."[2] They certainly thought of themselves as intellectuals, as were fellow scientists Ernst Rutherford, Arthur Eddington, and the others, who pondered metaphysical as well as physical problems. But the new way that the term "intellectual" was being used was apparently dismissive of natural scientists' mental endeavors. Intellectual came to mean "literary intellectual", those who were non-scientists and who, according to Snow, thought that scientists were "unaware of man's condition," whereas, in response, scientists considered literary types to be introspective and "lacking in foresight."[1]

Suddenly, scientists were seen as out of touch with the human condition, an irony since science so powerfully impacted humanity through developments in the physical sciences. And yet what surprised Snow and his friends was that the history of science was full of examples of scientists engaged in deep philosophical thought about their work, hence being referred to as natural philosophers before the neologism 'scientist' appeared in the 1830s. Even more surprising is that another branch of science, medical science, was similarly being seen as increasingly distant from the humanities throughout the twentieth century. In this uncertain space, between the laboratories and the waiting rooms of concerned and confused patients, emerged a now common feature of medical education programs called the "Medical Humanities."

I am the director of one such Medical Humanities program, in the School of Medicine at UCSF. I know from first hand experience that many people see the term as a juxtaposition—they don't see the relevance of the humanities, with its concern for history, creative writing, poetry, or the visual arts, as relevant to the science and practice of medicine. These people make my life difficult. But then there are others who think the term is redundant, since (to paraphrase the physician and philosopher Edmund Pellegrino) medicine is the most humane of the sciences, if also the most scientific of the humanities. If there is an irony here, it is in the idea that the healing arts of medicine need a sub-discipline to somehow connect them with humanity.

I put forward these thoughts as a way of historicizing the alleged duality of the so-called "two cultures" of science and the humanities to ask, in a general way, what is the broader impact of this entire conference imagined to be, and more specifically, what relevance does the privileged reading we have had from Philip Levine have to occupational and environmental health. More bluntly, why should we be listening to poetry?

As you may presuppose, I get this sort of question nearly every week, because in my classes, medical students not only read but they try to write poetry. Sometimes we talk about it as a means of improving communication skills, but that is a diversionary tactic, to get people to think about a "skill set" rather than the meaning of what we are doing. More truthfully, it is a means of promoting self-reflection and critical intellectual engagement with their own feelings. We intellectualize feelings in order to make them more appropriate to the context of university education. But we are also reconnecting with a practice common to medical men and women for a very long time. Whatever the alleged distance between medicine and the humanities today, medicine itself has a very rich literary culture, and therefore Philip Levine's relevance is not only intellectual, but historical.

Think about physician writers. Rabelais, Tobias Smollett, Erasmus Darwin, John Keats, Oliver Wendell Holmes, Arthur Conan Doyle, Anton Chekhov, A.J. Cronin, and William Carlos Williams. More recently we have writers like Richard Selzer writing about rituals of surgery, Raphael Campo, and our own resident physician poet here at UCSF David Watts, besides hundreds of others who publish poems, short stories, and books about life, medicine, the human condition and the ways to condition our humanity. The language of medicine is complex, but never more so than when it grapples with the fundamental anxieties we all share—whether physicians, patients, or poets—about the two cultures of life and death. Literature, non-fiction or fiction, prose or poetry, provides us with a way of thinking about and communicating these concerns amongst ourselves in ways that science cannot.

If medical science is an impenetrable matrix of technical jargon and unpronounceable terms to the lay public, then it is all the more important that the humanities provide people with a means of communicating about their condition, their lives, the contexts of their concerns. As Levine wrote in his poem Detroit Grease Shop, "We're all here to count and be counted", and craftsmen of words like him help make sure that everyone is included in that metric.

The relevance of engaging with expressions borne from the fields of the humanities to our understanding of medicine and healthcare should be apparent. And while I again suggest that it is a cliché that we live in "two cultures" of science and literature, it is worth being historically accurate and noting that C.P. Snow himself was *not* suggesting two such separate cultures, but rather one common concern that can be contemplated using the tools both of science and literature. Interestingly, it was when he starting thinking about medicine that CP Snow offered his clearest example of this complementarity. In a short piece published in *JAMA*, Snow wrote:[3]

> We have all known physicians who are wise, we have known some who are wise and have learned nothing from books, we have known some, in fact, who are wise and nearly illiterate. I want to suggest to you that they would

> have been a shade wiser with the elements of a humanistic education. You can't teach wisdom, you certainly cannot teach empathy, yet if the potentiality of empathy exists in anyone, then it can be encouraged by those who have possessed it, and have tried to express it in words. That is why I am inclined to think that there ought to be a literary component throughout the course of medical education. That is a practical example of what I meant when I spoke about the two cultures.

Science and medicine have much to learn from the humanities, and vice versa. History, literature and poetry provide ways of communicating that can be both insightful of conditions affecting our wellbeing as well as therapeutic to how we cope with these conditions. And in these ways it is all the more important that we celebrate the achievements of humanists like Philip Levine and listen carefully to the voices of those he brings to our notice through his work.

References

1 C.P. Snow, *The Two Cultures and the Scientific Revolution: The Rede Lecture 1959* (Cambridge: Cambridge University Press, 1959), p. 4, p. 6.

2 G.H. Hardy, *A Mathematician's Apology* (Cambridge: Cambridge University Press, 1940), p. 10.

3 C.P. Snow, Letter to the Editor, *JAMA* (1973) 225, pp. 619.

Made in the USA
Monee, IL
04 November 2026

67385947R10134